Bon Bons to YOGA PANTS

Bon Bons to YOGA PANTS

Katie Cross

Antebellum
Publishing

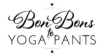

YOGA to PANTS

Contemporary ChickLit

Text copyright ©2015 by Katie Cross

Cover designed by Jenny Zemanek at www.seedlingsonline.com
Typesetting by Chris Bell with Atthis Arts LLC at www.atthisarts.com
Ebook formatting by Kella Campbell with Ebooks Done Right at www.ebooksdoneright.com

Published by Antebellum Publishing.
Visit www.antebellumpublishing.com for more information.

ISBN (paperback) 978-0-9966249-0-9
(ebook) 978-0-9966249-1-6

Visit the author at www.kcrosswriting.com

Visit The Health and Happiness Society Series at www.healthandhappinesssociety.com or on Facebook at www.facebook.com/healthandhappinesssociety

To all the Lexies.

Author's Notes

Bon Bons to Yoga Pants (BBtYP) started out on Wattpad as a serial. I posted twice a week just for fun. It was my *author playground* if you will, a story that I didn't really have to plot out, but could take in bite-size pieces one chapter at a time. Every Monday and Thursday morning I would sit down, open Wattpad, and start writing whatever I felt needed to come next in Lexie's life. About an hour later, I'd post the chapter.

For a free-spirited creative like myself, BBtYP became a necessary escape from the outlines and greater editing that come with my fiction works.

I'm publishing BBtYP because it's a story that gained a lot more traction than I expected, and at a much greater rate. Several loyal Wattpad fans have requested that I offer it in print or as an ebook, and I'm only too happy to oblige. Beyond those considerations, I know that Lexie is a story that needs to be told.

Because of BBtYP's unusual origins as an online serial, it's something of a different setup. The scenes are more or less complete in themselves and are all about the same size and word count. They all contribute to the greater structure of the story, but also have more of a micro-plot than I would do in my typical fiction. The writing is more raw because I felt the topic and nature of Lexie's story deserved the natural state. Except for copy edits to catch mistakes and proofreading to catch even more mistakes, the only real editing that occurred in this story is my own. In that way, Lexie is the most authentic voice I can give you.

Lexie is a girl born out of the depths of my own experiences and past. She is a person I have been, will be, and will always hold close to my heart. More than that, she is every person in some way, whether we are short, tall, thin, or overweight. Lexie's journey is more than just weight loss; it's coming to terms with who we are fundamentally, and learning that self-worth doesn't depend on jean size, whether we feel we are too big or too small.

Going through this journey with her was freeing, heartbreaking, and incredibly fun. It will remain as one of my favorite experiences as an author, and will always have a special place in my heart.

I hope you enjoy Lexie as much as I have.

Chapter 1—An Eternal Question

Like any great story, it all began with Facebook.

"Stupid internet," I muttered, slamming my desk drawer shut, as if that would help my Facebook profile load faster. The internet had an attitude and decided to pretend it was dial-up. The connection had definitely frozen. "How am I supposed to stalk Bradley if the internet won't even work?"

Behind me came the everyday sounds of my mom getting ready upstairs. Light chitter-chatter, the smell of coffee beans, and a shriek when my younger sister McKenzie realized she'd missed a text message from her fiancé.

"Finally!" I cried under my breath, exultant when the eternal rainbow of death stopped spinning and opened my profile page. My eyes immediately zipped to the notification bar, and I felt a little twinge of hope when I saw a red number.

Four notifications.

My heart sped up. It had to be Bradley, my secret online lovecrush. It just had to be. With a trembling hand I sent the arrow to the right spot, clicked, and brought up the screen. My heart sank.

The notification wasn't from Bradley. Neither was the message, which was actually from my sister McKenzie, who lived exactly two stories above me and still texted or messaged me when she had a question. The last thing I wanted to read was a message from an annoying twit who flounced her massive engagement ring around. Besides, I already knew what it was going to say.

How's the diet going? You didn't send me your calorie count yesterday. My July wedding is only six months away, remember?

Fabulous, I would respond. *That new calorie counting app you sent me is great. I'll send you my numbers.*

Then I'd eat another cinnamon roll just because she couldn't see me from my basement lair and send her fake numbers.

I shut the web browser with an angry click, feeling as if I'd exacted my vengeance on McKenzie for her prying and Bradley for . . . well,

1

nothing. Yet. He would come through. I'd uploaded a new profile picture onto Facebook last night. It had been a good one, albeit older, taken at least a year—or three—before. The photo was neck up, of course, because otherwise Mom and McKenzie would say something about my lack of weight loss.

Such a pretty face, I heard Mom say in the back of my head. *But let's go for a walk and get some exercise, shall we?*

Bradley had said he wanted to see a picture of my face, which was fair, because I had already seen plenty of pictures of his beautiful, beautiful face. Chocolate brown hair, hazel eyes, and a killer smile that belonged on the cover of *GQ.* I shook my head and slipped into a favorite pair of sweat pants. McKenzie would roll her eyes and say, *You're wearing those again?*

Today was my lucky day, however, as the door slammed twice within the same minute, leaving me alone in a blissfully quiet house. I threw on my sports bra, pulled on my hoodie, and put my hair into a ponytail. Why get dressed up for an early morning statistics class?

Once I stepped into the kitchen, I drew in a deep breath and then let it all out again with a contented sigh. *My haven.* How wonderful was the kitchen? So stable, so solid. It never asked me, *do you have enough calories left today to eat that second ravioli?* Or judged me when I had leftover pizza for breakfast because I was in too much of a hurry for my next class to cook the fat free turkey bacon that McKenzie insisted was healthy.

I was a college sophomore. Marinara sauce should have been in my blood, right?

Eating breakfast without Mom around to eye my portion sizes was a rare treat, so I stocked up with a double size helping of cereal and turned on an old episode of *The Golden Girls* to start my day. Mom didn't even know I had cold cereal. I laughed with wicked delight.

A note on the fridge door stopped me as I reached for the milk, already dreaming of eating the crunchy sweetness.

Don't forget to meet us at the bridal shop at 3. Your dress came in. And it BETTER fit.

—*Kenz*

With a sigh, I crumpled the note in my fist, tossed it down the garbage disposal, and rooted through my hidden stash of cereal behind the garbage bags on the top shelf. Dad had never cared about my weight, so why were Mom and Kenzie always on my case? An eternal question. A twinge of longing struck my heart.

Too bad Dad wasn't here anymore.

Besides, it wasn't like I was *that* overweight. I could still fit into sweat pants. Jeans were uncomfortable anyway because they restricted movement, or that's what I told myself. Hoodies hid most of my waist. As long as I didn't wear my hair down on my shoulders, my face looked thin enough. Despite the strength of my denial, in the end, I knew my mom and sister were right. Two hundred and fifty pounds didn't hide easily.

Oh, how I wish it did.

Chapter 2—Bloated Flamingo

The bridesmaid dress made me look like a bloated flamingo.

Three mirrors reflecting my rolling hips and thighs didn't help. My size eighteen hips and less-than-impressive chest formed a perfect oval next to McKenzie's lithe, size-four, hourglass figure.

"This is what you picked out? Seriously?" I asked, running my fingers over the silky material. Kenz flittered around me, squealing with delight.

"Oh!" she squeaked. "It's perfection!"

If an overstuffed bottle of Pepto-Bismol was perfect, then yes, I looked perfect.

"Mom—" I began.

"Just a second, honey," she said, waving an absent hand through the air while fidgeting with a pink bow at my side. A sales lady in a svelte black suit hovered just behind Mom like a storm cloud, no doubt sensing the inevitable sale. Mom never could prevent herself from buying anything pink. I rolled my eyes, let out a dramatic sigh, and then glanced at the clock.

Salvation!

"Oh look at the time!" I cried, "Gotta get to work."

Mom opened her mouth to protest, a deep wrinkle forming on her forehead. She must have caught a reflection of herself on one of the mirrors because she instantly straightened her forehead and let the wrinkle smooth out. She was an attractive, lean woman with streaks of gray in her blonde hair, cut into a tasteful bob. Except for McKenzie's deep brown hair, which she'd gotten from Dad, the two of them could have been twins.

"Well, at least we know the dress fits and looks . . . lovely," Mom said. I ignored her hesitation.

"I love it!" McKenzie's squeaky girl voice mimicked the tiny mouse of her body. "It'll go just great with all the pink azaleas. You could lose a few pounds, you know Lexie, and it would fit better."

She put her hands on her hips and set a determined eye on me.

"Gotta go," I said, stepping off the stand of death, ducking away

4

from the bright lights, and stumbling into the back dressing room. After peeling off the dress that fit like a banana skin, I returned to the comfortable relief of my usual clothes and slung my backpack over my shoulder.

McKenzie's lower lip stuck out in a mock pout when I emerged.

"Not that old outfit again," she muttered, rolling her eyes. "You look like you're on your way to the gym, not work."

I ignored her, kissed Mom on the cheek, and called a farewell over my shoulder. A blast of cold, snowy air met me with a cool kiss on my flushed cheeks.

Pink for a bridesmaid, I thought with a grimace, heading down the hazy street. *I'll have to work overtime to make sure Bradley doesn't see any pictures of it on Facebook.*

I pulled my phone out of the side pocket of my backpack. No messages. No notifications. With a sigh I threw it back into the pocket and zipped it closed. He must have been busy today. I normally heard from him by now.

McKenzie's admonishment to lose weight accompanied me to Lucky's, the Irish pub where I'd worked since graduating high school. Most nights I wore a white t-shirt and hid behind a green apron with a shamrock on front. Most customers didn't notice me when they ordered, just the way I liked it.

My boss Pat stood behind a long cherry wood bar when I walked in, setting the bell jangling, and inhaling the familiar scent of yeast and cloves. Pat was a round man with bright apple cheeks and a smile that made his eyes disappear. He waved and continued speaking with a guy at the opposite end of the bar.

"Sorry I was almost late!" I called. "Mom stuffed me into a pink thing that made it look like a Smurf vomited."

As usual, business was never busy at the pub during the late afternoon on a weekday. After ensuring the glasses were clean, the bar wiped, and no one needed anything, I opened my homework beneath the lip of the bar, keeping my phone where I could see it in case Bradley texted me, and set to my homework.

Twenty minutes later, the bell announced a new customer.

"Hey Mira," Pat said, averting his eyes. His cheeks flared an even brighter red. "Thanks for coming."

"Hullo, Pat," she called. My mom's best friend, Mirabelle, shoved a chair out of her way and slapped a pamphlet on the bar in front of me. She wore an outlandish, wide-brimmed hat with a bird nesting in hay. The bright red ribbon around it matched her lipstick, which smeared her face. She wore a roomy muumuu dress that made her look like a walking blue blob.

"Do it with me," she said, meeting my startled gaze. "I'm supposed to take a friend."

I glanced at the flyer, which showed a picture of an exercise ball and a set of weights, and then back to her.

"What is it?" I asked. Exercise equipment? This couldn't be good.

"It's a dieting group."

"What?" I screeched. "What kind of dieting group?"

Mira straightened up, tilting her hat back so it didn't shade her eyes.

"The kind that helps you diet," she replied, whipping the pamphlet open and pointing to a cluster of words in the middle. "They meet every Wednesday night. That's your night off. You're coming."

I laughed and pushed it away. "I don't need to join a dieting group."

"Yes, you do."

My eyes narrowed on her. "That's pretty rude."

She glanced down to the plate of sausage and cabbage that Pat had fixed for me, back to me, and then to the plate again. A noise came out of the back of her throat, and my narrowed eyes became a sharp glare of warning.

No *way* would she start taking away my food.

"Your sister is getting married. Both of us could stand to lose a few pounds for the wedding."

"So?"

"Your Mama told me that your dress is skintight."

I gasped. "You went to my mom? Traitor! You know how she is about my weight."

She straightened her neck with a haughty sniff. "Of course I did. I had to make it happen, didn't I? I stopped by the bridal shop just before I came here."

Mira and Mom had been best friends since they were five. When

Mira's husband died of a heart attack two years ago, she'd fallen into piles of food for comfort and gained fifty pounds. I'd been there to help her through many pints of Ben and Jerry's, sharing my own grief for losing Dad while she mourned her husband.

"Mira, I don't have time for this. Think of all my homework! I have to have three books read and analyzed by the end of the week."

"Read while you work out."

"I can't afford gym fees."

"I'm buying."

"Healthy food is expensive."

"Your mom is the healthiest person I know," she said with a roll of her eyes. "You live at home with both her and McKenzie. You have no lack of healthy food."

My nostrils flared. Drat! Out of excuses. Before I could come up with a really good reason this wouldn't work, she pulled out the Big One.

"Don't you want to meet Bradley with confidence?" She fluttered her eyelashes in an innocent way. "I imagine he'll want to meet you in person soon."

I glowered at her. Except for my best friend Rachelle, Mira was the only person on earth that knew I'd met Bradley online and had been conversing for several months.

"That's not fair. Besides, I'm never going to meet Bradley. We have an online thing going. That's the beauty of it. He never has to see what I actually look like."

"Life isn't fair. You know that already. Don't you want to be happy, Lex?"

The feeling of changing into the bridesmaid dress not even an hour before replayed through my mind. Miserable. It made me totally miserable, not happy. The glum realization that I couldn't remember the last time I *had* felt happy came to me with striking force.

But surely I wasn't so big that Mira needed to force me into losing weight.

Was I?

Or did I just live in a world of denial so I didn't have to see the truth?

As if she'd read my mind, Mira said in a quiet, understanding voice, "It's not about your size, honey. Not really. You're perfect the way you are no matter how much you weigh. It's about being healthy. It's about being strong and in control. It's about being happy again . . ."

The distant, teary look in her eyes broke my building resistance. How could I say no? Mira might as well have been my mother—she understood me far better than my own mother did—and I couldn't bear to see her so sorrowful.

I drew in a deep breath and looked to the warm, delicious plate of food beneath me. Why hadn't I at least scarfed the bread down before I started my homework?

"Fine," I muttered, pushing the plate away. "I'll do it."

She beamed, nearly knocking her hat off. "I thought you would, honey. I thought you would."

Chapter 3—Operation Meet Bradley

♠

How was the day?

Bradley's message popped up on my Facebook screen the moment I logged in. My heart spasmed with joy. After such a long day, his profile picture was exactly what I needed to see. I dropped my heavy backpack, tossed my notebook on top of my desk, and fell into the chair.

Busy, I replied, my keyboard clacking as my fingers danced across the keys. Light from the computer screen illuminated my face in the dark basement. *My sister made me try on my bridesmaid dress for the first time. *barf**

While waiting for his response, I reached for the microwave burrito I'd warmed up for dinner, since I'd sacrificed my usual dinner at the pub to the gods of dieting. I stared at the warm tortilla with a twinge of guilt. McKenzie's voice in the back of my head reminded me that these burritos had at least 700 calories.

Which explained why they were oh-so-addicting.

Wasn't a normal adult female allowed three thousand calories or something like that? Besides, I hadn't eaten since lunch and my stomach growled in ravenous hunger.

"Last hurrah," I promised myself, and tore into the cheesy beans with a destructive first bite. Bradley's typing indicator popped up while I chewed through three massive mouthfuls.

Is the dress as pink as she threatened? he asked.

Pinker. Think Pepto-Bismol meets Barbie.

Sisters, calories, and diets aside, Bradley had been my best friend for the last two months. When Ben and Jerry just didn't comfort me, his online attention and subtle emoticons saved the day. My favorite part? Crushing on him from afar without the horror of meeting him in person and making a fool of myself.

The clock on my computer said 10:30 pm, and I still had homework. The temptation to close our conversation and finish my homework so I could sleep flickered through me, but I sent it away with a scoff. Bradley brightened my day. I'd stay up until three in the morning talking to him if he wanted. We'd certainly done it before.

Well, I hope to see you in it at her wedding, he said. *Sounds pretty epic.*

My eyes widened and I dropped the half-eaten burrito onto my lap. Bradley had never broached the topic of meeting in person. Our Facebook friendship had magic because I built it on dreams that involved nothing with reality. I blinked three times, completely derailed. Meet Bradley in person?

Unsure of how to play it cool, I simply responded with: *?*

The typing indicator seemed to last forever before his reply came.

My friend is moving out there, and he needs someone to help him drive, so I volunteered. He's moving into a place about an hour from your town. I thought it would be the perfect opportunity for us to finally meet up.

My heart pounded.

Yeah, of course! I wrote at first, then backspaced. No exclamation point. I needed to play this *very* cool. *Yeah, of course. I'll need a date for the wedding anyway.*

I hit return before I'd even thought of how my response it sounded. As soon as the words appeared in the chat screen, I screamed.

"No!"

Too late. I'd put the words into cyberspace forever. "Oh no!" I moaned. "He's totally going to think I asked him out."

Ages passed before his response came.

That sounds awesome. Consider it a date. Listen, I need to go study. I'll chat with you later.

He left.

I stared at the computer screen in mute shock. Had I scared him away? Was it really going to be awesome?

Really?

I glanced down to see the burrito sitting in my lap, cheese spewing out like refried lava. My eyes trailed to my less-than-muscular thighs, my chubby fingers, and finally to my ample stomach. He didn't know what I looked like! He didn't know that I wore hoodies and flip-flops because I hated my body.

My eyes fell on my notebook. A corner of Mirabelle's pamphlet stuck out from the bottom page. With great reluctance, I tugged it loose.

Join us Wednesday nights at 6:00 pm.

Changing your life starts now!

I glanced back to the computer screen, down to the half-spilled burrito in my lap, and finally up to the picture of Dad I'd taped to my computer screen. He had a round, full face just like me. He'd been overweight and unhappy.

Just like me.

Mira's voice floated back through my mind.

It's about being healthy. It's about being strong and in control. It's about being happy again . . .

I drew in a deep, resolute breath.

"All right," I said to Dad, tossing the burrito into my garbage can. "It's on. I have six months to lose weight. Operation Meet Bradley begins tonight."

Chapter 4—Health and Happiness Society

"**Welcome to the first** official meeting of the *Health and Happiness Society*. Mira is passing around a tray of ice water. Feel free to drink all you want because it's calorie free."

A woman named Bitsy stood at the top of the room in a pair of tight black workout capris, a baggy shirt, and her hair in a messy bun. She had the air of a frazzled mom that hadn't had the time to lose the baby weight. I silently applauded her moxie at wearing form-fitting pants; I'd never be caught dead in such a tight set of trousers. I secretly envied the girls who could wear yoga pants. If I tried, my legs had enough unattractive lumps and bumps that it would look like someone stuffed marshmallows down my pants

Mira shoved a glass of ice water into my hands. "Take it and drink up," she said. "I hear ice water increases your metabolism."

Unable to refuse because she'd probably dump it in my lap, I took the sweating, cold glass and had a sip. Plain water sounded as appetizing as dry broccoli. It needed a good scoop of lemonade powder. My lips pursed just thinking of the tart and sweet flavor.

Delish.

"Thank you for coming tonight and taking time out of your busy lives to take care of your health," Bitsy continued, as if our losing weight benefitted her in some personal endeavor. "Trust me when I say that the investment is worth it."

The couch I sat on was scratchy and old, in a living room filled with odd trinkets and a small TV. Several pictures of two young girls playing with a dark-haired man littered the walls, although I didn't see Bitsy in any of them. An impressive number of Jillian Michaels workout DVDs were stacked on a rack. It wasn't the most up-to-date house, but it was certainly spotless.

Four other people filled the room, the first of the *Health and Happiness Society*. Bitsy, our fearless and somewhat drill sergeant-esque leader, Mira, myself, and two men who sat on opposite sides of the room. Every age, height, and weight seemed to have representation. The only thing we appeared to have in common was one obvious trait: we all were a little soft around the edges.

Okay, a lot soft. Around *all* edges.

"This group is a support group," Bitsy explained. "We'll weigh in before every meeting and report our calorie intake for the week. Don't worry! Your weigh-in will be totally confidential. Just between you and me. Then as a group we'll discuss what we've struggled with that week and do a recipe swap."

Mira had finished passing around the water, and now handed out pieces of paper. I felt like I'd just walked into an AA meeting.

Hi, I pictured myself saying. *My name is Lexie, and all I can think about right now is chicken pad thai.*

The handout contained a brief overview of dieting strategies. Nothing I hadn't heard before, of course. Mom had me on a diet since high school, when she first started to notice my pants filling out. She'd panicked and threatened to put me on a diet of only grapefruit and cucumber water. Thankfully, Mira had talked her out of it. Dad had just laughed it off and reached for another glazed doughnut saying, "She's got some meat on her bones, that's all!"

Don't shop on an empty stomach, the paper preached. *Fill up with a glass of water before dinner.* And, my personal favorite, *don't eat when you're feeling emotional.*

I snorted. Fat chance.

Mira sat next to me, the scent of lavender drifting behind her like a trailing wind.

"Don't look so angry," she whispered, shooting me a sharp look of disapproval. "No one will want to be your friend, and you shouldn't diet alone. They say that you're 75% more likely to lose weight when you do it as part of a group."

While I doubted she quoted actual statistics, I didn't have a chance to call her out on it. One of the men on the other side of the room stood up, his hands fidgeting nervously in front of an impressive beer belly. He had a shiny, bald head underneath his greasy comb-over, and a wide pair of coke bottle glasses.

"Hi," he said, clearing his throat. "I'm Ken."

"Hi Ken," Bitsy and Mira echoed, as if they operated from one brain.

"I'm a father of five. I lost my job last year and turned to food for comfort. I want to lose weight again because I don't like myself anymore and I'm depressed. I also want to live to see my grandkids."

He paused, as if he wanted to say more, then sat down.

I hear you, brother, I wanted to say. *Food is the greatest comfort. It never lets me down. Especially egg rolls with sweet and sour dipping sauce.*

The introductions moved around the room one at a time until all their eyes landed on me. The moment I felt the power of their stares, I pulled my hoodie out to make sure it wasn't sticking to my rolling stomach and slowly stood.

"I'm Lexie," I said with an awkward wave. "I want to lose 100 pounds because there's a guy I want to date."

The two men nodded politely, but clearly couldn't care less. Bitsy, however, honed her sharp eyes on me like a hawk.

"Is that the only reason?" she asked.

We stared at each other for a tense moment. She was definitely the kind of woman who lived in Mom mode and snapped out commands like a four star general.

"Oh, yeah," I added, realizing that she wanted more from me. "And for my health and stuff."

She lifted an eyebrow; I certainly hadn't fooled her. Instead of calling me out for being a superficial college student who would only meet with failure *because beauty comes from within,* she simply smiled in a terse way.

"Well, welcome to the *Health and Happiness Society,* Lexie. We're glad to have you. Just as soon as Mira introduces herself, we'll go into the back for the weigh-in, and figure out from there what everyone's daily calorie allotment should be."

My sigh of relief stopped.

Wait.

Calorie allotment?

Couldn't I just cut down my portion sizes and call it good? That's what I'd done today. I had just one sandwich at lunch instead of two. My stomach kept growling and I couldn't think of anything but food, which meant the diet must already be working. Couldn't I just weigh myself and not have anyone else know how high the scale had been creeping?

Bradley's new photo on Facebook that morning flashed through my mind. He was so beautiful, with the sculpted planes of his Greek god face. My eyes drifted down to my too-big scrub pants and overly large baggy sweatshirt. I couldn't risk meeting Bradley wearing a hoodie. Surely he wouldn't be attracted to me, Lexie Greene, college student and certified bartender.

No, I had to do it. I had to count calories and . . . weigh in.

I let out a long breath and steeled myself for what would surely be the most depressing reckoning I'd had in months.

The scale.

Chapter 5—The Scale Room

The Scale Room was an overstuffed bathroom with pictures of kids dressed up like flowers. A basket of toys hung over the side of the bathtub, a bowl of stale potpourri sat on the back of the toilet, and entirely too much baby blue wallpaper filled the walls. The theme for *Jaws* played in the back of my mind when I stepped inside. There was barely enough room for me and Bitsy both, which made me feel even more awkward. What was I supposed to do with my hands? I opted for tucking them in the pouch of my sweatshirt.

Perfect. Cover up that stomach.

"Just step right on the scale," Bitsy said, motioning with a tilt of her head to the square of doom on the floor. She scribbled something on an old clipboard, and I hesitated.

"Can I take off my shoes?"

"Sure."

On and on she wrote, increasing my paranoia with every second. Was she recording state secrets? Was my weight going to be one of them? I shucked off my tennies and wished I'd worn something besides the heavy sweatshirt. I could deduct ten pounds just taking that off, no doubt. I stared at the scale, mentally preparing for the inevitable wave of self-loathing that accompanied every weight measurement. What a particularly heartless foe the scale could be.

As if she smelled weakness, Bitsy glanced up at me, one eyebrow arched so high it almost touched her brown hair.

"Well?"

"I need to prepare myself." I let out a long breath. "Do I have to see the number?"

"You don't *have* to do anything, but I highly recommend that you face your starting point. It can be very motivational when you don't want to work out, or when the doughnut calls. And trust me; they will call."

Doughnuts and I had such a good relationship these days that they didn't even call anymore; they walked right in the open door of my mouth. Just thinking about pastries made my mouth water. Apple fritters were my favorite. They had that sweet glaze on top that had just a hint of—

"Stop daydreaming about doughnuts," she snapped. "You can't put this off forever, Lex."

Lex? I wanted to say, annoyed. Since when did we start chatting on a nickname basis? And how did she know what I was thinking about?

"Right," I muttered, cracking my knuckles. "I can do this."

My heart skipped a beat as I stepped on her uber-expensive, from-the-future scale that analyzed everything except DNA coding. I stared at the wall, my heart in my throat.

"Okay," Bitsy said, fingers flying across the clipboard. "259."

"What?" I screeched, my eyes bugging out of my face. "When did I gain 10 pounds?"

"When did you last weigh?"

"I don't know," I mumbled, stepping off the scale. "Few months ago."

"You were at 249?"

"Ish," I hedged, met her expectant stare, and capitulated with a sigh. "245."

Bitsy said nothing about my purposefully terrible math skills. Having only ten extra pounds sounded so much better than fourteen, but it didn't matter. I always rounded down.

"Can I take off a few pounds for my clothes?" I asked hopefully. "Oh, and it's the end of the day! This is all water weight and stuff, right?"

Bitsy shook her head. "No. Your clothes don't weigh a couple of pounds, Lex. Sorry."

The shame hurt. 259.

My highest *ever*.

"You're inactive, right?" she asked, unaware that what little self-esteem I had writhed in agony on the floor.

"Inactive?"

"Do you work out?"

I snorted. *Jab that fat girl knife in a little deeper, Bits.*

"I'll take that as a no . . ." she drawled, her eyes back on the clipboard. I sat on the toilet and tried to imagine myself in a happy place. Chipotle. Eating a burrito. With avocado and the corn salsa that had just enough spice but not too—

"Based on my calculations," Bitsy said, continuing in true drill-master style, "in order to lose roughly a pound of weight a week, you may consume no more 1,800 calories per day. I'd probably consume at least 1,500 while starting. There are several apps you can use on your phone to track every single bite of food you take. *Everything*. Or you can write it down the old fashioned way, I don't care either way. Then, when you report back next week, I want you to tell me how many calories you burned each day, and how many you consumed."

The burrito of my dreams popped.

"1,800 calories?"

My sister had given me a similar number, but I hadn't actually looked at the dieting outline she'd drawn up on my behalf. All I saw was *Lexie's Diet Plan* written across the pages and tuned it out with a visit to my best friend, Little Debbie.

"It's more than some of us get," Bitsy said with forced cheer. "I'll be living on 1,300 calories."

"Is that humanly possible?" I asked, stumbling back into my shoes, fairly confident I could nom 1,300 calories at breakfast.

"Yes. I've done it plenty of times."

Plenty of times? What did that even mean? Was I doomed to a lifestyle of continual dieting and perpetual self-hatred on the scale? She read my mind again.

"Don't be discouraged, Lexie. It's good to face down your demons and hit rock bottom. Then you have nowhere else to go but up."

No, sister, I wanted to say. *I've seen rock bottom when Dad died, and it's littered with sugary treats.*

"Right," I retorted. "Don't be discouraged."

Was she kidding? Not only was I now on a diet that *didn't* involve Fruit Loops, but I had fifteen more pounds to lose than I thought! Visions of dinner started to dance through my head like sugarplums in the old Christmas poem. I'd find comfort in French bread and lasagna.

"Don't do it," Bitsy said, reaching for the door handle, her sharp eye on me. I reared back.

"What?"

"I know that look. You want to go home and eat to make yourself feel better. That's the last thing you should do."

I cleared my throat. Bitsy was getting downright *freaky.* "Of course not. I was going to . . . go for a walk, or something."

Ha! I hadn't been on a walk since I was fifteen.

She studied my face, her lips pinched and eyes narrowed. Her kids were probably perfect angels; no human soul would dare misbehave with a look like that coming at them.

"You can do this, Lexie," she said, pulling the door open. "But it's going to be hell. Just embrace it and push through the suck."

I followed on her heels out of the close, overly pastel blue bathroom with relief.

It's going to be hell. Just embrace it.

The only thing I wanted in my embrace was a jelly doughnut.

Chapter 6—Old-Fashioned Bradley

Hey. How was your day?

Bradley's message came to my phone, since I was studying at my desk with my computer purposefully turned off to avoid social media. But I couldn't be *too* disconnected because . . . Bradley.

I glanced at the littered remnants of my post-Health-and-Happiness-Society-meeting snack with shame. Although I'd opted for the healthier option of yogurt tubes and bologna—probiotics and protein, obviously—I still felt ashamed of the food binge. Bitsy would go berserk, no doubt. Probably blow a whistle in my face. Even justifying the mad binge by saying that I hadn't tracked calories for anything else today so why start at nine o'clock didn't make it seem any better.

"Tomorrow," I said in a poor attempt at consoling myself. "The calorie count begins."

Just to prove I meant it, I downloaded the calorie counting app that Bitsy recommended in her pamphlet.

Oh, I finally responded to Bradley in the chat window. *Today was just . . . peachy.*

Doesn't sound good.

It was fine, just a meeting that didn't go quite the way I wanted. How about you?

Just got home from a date.

My gut clenched. Of course he did! That's what normal people did on a Wednesday, right? I let out a heavy sigh, not certain I wanted to hear the details. But he seemed to enjoy hashing his dates out with me afterwards, like some kind of therapy for PTSD or something.

At least, that's what *I* always needed after dates. Okay, I'd only been on two dates, and both had been horrible experiences. I swallowed my pride. If Bradley wanted to talk about his date, that was fine with me. I'd talk to him about almost anything.

Almost. I wasn't about to dive into a conversation about how difficult it was to find comfortable jeans in my size these days.

How did it go? I asked.

He took his time responding. Probably fielding off future dates or saving a kitten.

Nothing magical with this date. There rarely is anymore. :(

A smile crept across my face. He was so cute sometimes! Just when I started to get annoyed, he always said something so adorable I could have vomited rainbows.

And you're expecting magic? I asked.

Definitely.

I sighed. I couldn't help it. I was just girly enough to still believe in the ridiculous Cinderella dreams of my childhood. The kind where Prince Charming rode in on a white horse, where the dress always fit, and the hair curled in messy perfection. Never mind that I'd never fit in a glass slipper. I couldn't even buy boots to fit over my calves.

That's a rare trait to find in a guy. I unwittingly fell into daydreams of Bradley riding up on his powerful stallion, his hair ruffled by the wind, strong arms held out, waiting for me to . . .

Startled from my reverie by the obnoxious chime that meant he'd responded, I jumped and my phone clattered to the floor. "I've reached a new level of pathetic," I mumbled, straightening my skewed glasses while scrambling to hold the phone upright again.

I get that about a lot of things, he said. *I'm too old fashioned.*

My eyebrows rose with interest. *Oh?* I asked. *What other things? Do tell.*

It's really not that interesting.

I'd be the better judge of that.

My heart beat in time with the cursor. He seemed to be typing forever before the response came.

I like being the guy in the relationship. Sometimes I feel like women are trying too hard to be the man. Tonight, this girl didn't even want me to open the door for her. Seriously? That's ridiculous. Does that sound stupid or anti-feminist? That's not what I meant by it. I've just dated women that have to control everything, even my part of the relationship, and it was miserable.

I read his response five times, less convinced every time that he was human, and not some machine inputted to know all the right responses.

"You can't be real," I finally concluded, my lips puckered to one side of my face. The hair fell from my loose bun that stood askew on top of my head. "Definitely can't be real. No one says that kind of crap anymore."

But his response seemed so sincere that I didn't know what to say. I growled and leaned back in my chair so I could stare at the glow-in-the-dark stars on my ceiling. Dad had helped me put the stars up when I first moved to the basement all by myself. "You'll never be lonely sleeping beneath the stars, Lex," he'd said.

When I didn't respond for a stretch of time, the three dots indicating Bradley was typing popped up.

Uh oh. Did I say something to insult you?

My thumb hovered above the screen of my phone.

No, I finally replied. *No, it's just that what you said sounds perfect. I suppose it took me by surprise.*

See? Rare trait. :)

But I certainly wasn't smiling. My eyes strayed over the litter of my four yogurt tubes—which were certainly too yummy to be allowed on my diet—and the empty package of bologna. With trepidation in my gut, I reviewed the calories printed on back.

"Gripes," I muttered, totaling the numbers in my head with a grimace. "And that was just a snack."

Well, Bradley said, *I need to get ready for class tomorrow. It's lab day. I'll talk to you tomorrow?*

Yes! Definitely. Tomorrow.

He signed off just in time for Mira to call. I reluctantly hit the "answer" button, closed my eyes, and let out a breathy, "Hey."

"You seemed upset when you left. Were you?"

"Heck yes! That weigh-in was awful."

"Reality is kind of a beast," Mira agreed, sounding depressed herself. "Talk to Bradley tonight?"

"A little bit."

When I didn't elaborate, she sighed. "What do you say to going to the gym with me in the morning?"

My eyes shot open. "The gym? Is that what you said? Can't be. W-where do you want to go?"

"The gym. You know . . . people go there to work out. Exercise and stuff."

I blinked twice, feeling a knot of anxiety in my chest. People watching me work out? My legs in tight black pants? Sweating in public? This reeked of eighth grade gym class humiliation all over again. I used to eat Fudge Rounds after class every day just to console myself. The cruel taunts of *that chubby girl* still pained me.

"I don't know, Mira. The gym? What if we walk around the block instead? While it's still dark, preferably. Walking is great exercise I hear. It's . . . aerobic or something."

"You don't even know what aerobic means."

"Not in regards to exercise, no."

"Nice try, but it's not happening," she drawled. "The gym it is. I've already paid for your membership. I'll be by at six, so don't be late."

The phone clicked and then buzzed with an empty line. Wily old Mira. She knew better than to give me a chance to make an excuse. I tossed my phone onto my bedspread and wilted into my chair. Bradley's saccharine-sweet conversation replayed in my head as if I'd actually heard him say the words, instead of just reading it.

"Fine," I said, smacking the armrest of my chair. "I'll go to the gym so I can be worthy of Bradley. I'll even count calories *and* go to the gym tomorrow."

No matter how much I tried to psyche myself up over it, the ugly truth couldn't be hidden.

The gym was going to be infinitely more humiliating than the scale.

Chapter 7—Gym Gazelles . . . er . . . Hippos

Mira charged into the gym as if she'd been there before. Which she hadn't, of course.

Never mind she was wearing a pair of bright blue sapphire leggings, a shirt so large that it hung to her knees, and a sweatband underneath a fluff of curly bangs. It had been years since I'd seen her without makeup, and her eyes seemed much smaller without exotic green eye shadow.

After checking in, she made a beeline straight for an elliptical, which I'd seen on TV before but never approached in person. I did so with the same hesitation I'd use to approach a ravenous bear just out of hibernation. *Exercise* outside of walking to and from my car was a bit of a foreign concept. I just didn't *do* stuff like this.

Anyway, most of the girls already gliding in place and glistening with moisture looked like gazelles. I, on the other hand, would look like a short-limbed hippo trying to fly.

"Mira, don't you think it's too early to work out?"

"Jump on!" she cried, jerking a thumb to the elliptical next to her. "They're low impact on your joints. We promised Bitsy we'd work out five times this week, remember?"

"No."

"It was in the contract you signed."

"I didn't sign a contract."

She smiled. "Oh, right. I signed it for you."

I surveyed my other options with dismay. Most machines looked as complicated as heart surgery, while the rest of the weight equipment obviously required a degree in ballet just to maneuver into the right position. The treadmill seemed safe except for one big problem . . . jiggle. My butt would wobble like jello salad with every step.

Deciding that the elliptical would indeed be the safest, I staggered over with dramatic flair.

Bradley *better* be worth it.

"You're supposed to work out early to kick start your metabolism,"

Mira said, moving her legs in an awkward, stiff rhythm on the smooth elliptical tracks. "If you don't eat before you work out, it's a double bonus! Look, I even brought you a water bottle. Staying hydrated is very important. Thirst is often mistaken as hunger."

She waved a Dasani in front of my face as if that were an incentive to be in a gym, surrounded by already fit people, at six in the morning. Water? She had to be kidding. Chocolate milk on the other hand . . .

I forced myself from the thought with a snap of my head. *Diet. Meeting Bradley. Looking hot.* I had objectives I *must* stick to. Oddly, the thought motivated me, so I climbed onto the hippo trap with very little grace.

"This better be worth it," I muttered under my breath, conjuring a daydream where I met Bradley. He, of course, looked perfect, with his warm smile and broad shoulders. A simple black dress for me, thanks. My hair would be longer by then, so I'd wear it up and—

An obnoxious beep from the machine broke into my happy reverie. I glanced down to see a myriad of flashing lights I didn't understand.

"Geez!" I pressed buttons, hoping it would stop alarming. "What did I do? Steal something?"

"You have to start it, silly," Mira said, reaching over to slap the *start* button. "You can configure your stats as you go."

"My stats?"

"Yeah, like age and weight. It figures out your calories from there. It's more accurate if you have a heartbeat monitor, of course." She thumped something underneath her shirt with a knuckle. "Then it's really accurate. I've already burned ten calories. I think that's a grape."

"Where do I insert my DNA and social security number?" I mumbled, but kept the roller legs going as I calmed the flashing words and input my numbers, not without some shame. After thorough study, and not a few muted swear words, the elliptical and I made peace with each other. For a while, it was nothing but smooth sailing and me in Bradley's embrace without an ounce of cottage cheese showing on the back of my arms.

"For Bradley," I reminded myself when the level increased and the top of my legs began to burn. "For Bradley."

Mira scowled. "For Lexie," she hissed. "You don't lose weight for a boy, silly girl. You do it for you, remember? *Health and Happiness Society*? Boys don't make you happy. Lexie makes Lexie happy."

Bradley's lips sure would make me happy, though.

"Oh, right," I agreed between pants. Mira shot me a suspicious glance, but returned to her TV program, and I returned to my Bradley fantasy. Or, more correctly, imagining the very moment he fell madly in love with me. The distraction of my daydream lasted for about ten minutes, and then I grew bored.

So bored that I sent a cursory glance to a table of magazines: *Elle. Vogue. Trail Running. Yeah, right,* I thought, snorting. *Like I want to look at what I will never be: a size zero model.* The news, a football re-run, or an old episode of *The Andy Griffith Show* were my only early morning options.

The most obvious choice remained—gym stalking.

Two college girls worked on bikes next to each other, textbooks in front of them, towels draped across their shoulders. How did legs that thin even move? Was that muscle, or straight bone? An Asian guy kept running past on the indoor track just in front of the elliptical, wheezing. Was that healthy? A guy with arms the size of a Christmas ham sat on a bench, elbow on his knee, curling a heavy weight while watching his bicep in the mirror. He seemed to fall in love with himself every time his veins bulged.

Free entertainment. Maybe this gym thing wouldn't be so bad.

Then my eyes caught onto something different. Two girls, their hair in braids, stood in the area of the gym reserved for weightlifters. Their ease in such a strange environment caught my attention. I couldn't stop staring, envying the way they seemed comfortable, not one bit afraid to be there. One glance confirmed it—they both wore tight black yoga pants.

"Whoa," I muttered as one girl, a brunette, reached for a heavy lifting bar stacked in the corner of the room. The other grabbed what seemed like an overabundance of heavy round weights and shoved them on the bar. The brunette positioned herself in front of the bar, squatted down, and began to lift it up and down. After ten, they switched.

I stopped spinning the elliptical to gawk. Were they *nuts?* Girls don't lift weights! That's a guy thing.

. . . Right?

By this point, Mira was moving so slowly while gaping at the TV overhead that the elliptical had shut off, erasing her programmed info.

What are we doing here? I thought, starting to move again when my elliptical squawked. I didn't belong in the gym, and Mira certainly didn't look at home either. Hippos in a group of prancing gazelles, that's what we were. Five minutes later my machine announced that my twenty minutes were up. I stepped off, except one foot was tangled in the other, the elliptical moved unexpectedly, and then . . . I fell.

With a smack.

Flat on my face.

Before I could really register what happened, a kind hand reached down and grabbed my arm, pulling me from my stumble.

"Hey, you all right?"

I gained my feet again with unusual speed for a girl my size, coming face to face with the brown eyes of the brunette girl I'd just been gym stalking and secretly envied.

"I'm good," I managed, with sheepish smile. "Thanks."

"Don't worry." She smiled, revealing a set of white teeth that had surely never known the metallic torture of braces. "I've fallen off them too. I hate those things. They're death traps."

For some reason, it made me feel better.

I should have been intimidated by her—because I usually would have been—but the feeling never came. She was neither skinny, nor fat. I couldn't even decide how to classify her, and I felt a burst of shame that I was even trying to. Wasn't there even solidarity amongst chubby girls?

"Thanks," I said, wanting to shake it off. "I appreciate the help."

One last smile and she was gone, walking to the water station for a drink. I watched her go. She wasn't perfect like the models in the magazines, but there was something about her that just seemed . . . great.

One day, I thought. *I want whatever it is that she's got.*

Shaking my head to clear my thoughts, I turned around to see Mira at a complete standstill, eyes riveted on a TV mystery drama with too many dark colors. At least she hadn't seen my disgrace.

"Come on, Mira," I said with a new burst of energy. "Let's try out the bikes, eh? We still have half an hour."

Chapter 8–Little Debbie is Not My Friend

To my deepest surprise, I didn't need to be taken out of the gym on a stretcher.

Except for when walking past an imprint of my face on the ground where I had fallen, I had a faint sense of accomplishment hidden in all the embarrassment. My legs were a bit wobbly, and my stomach revolted with constant demands to be fed, but I certainly didn't *die* the way I'd expected. While I didn't normally like the feeling of being sweaty, this wasn't the same kind of sweaty that I felt in the summer, when my body seemed to be drowning. This was a different sweat . . . a fresher kind.

I arrived home to an empty kitchen, and started the most serious business of my day: breakfast. But my hand stopped halfway to the usual go-to of breakfast sugar cereal. Although the crunchy sweet texture was surely what I wanted, my mind strayed back to the scale at Bitsy's house.

259

I sighed, dropped my arm, and reached for the fridge instead. No overly bright bowl of sugar for this girl. No doubt Kenzie would eat something healthy, based off broccoli or spinach instead of the reliable, processed goodness of cereal. I swiped a light yogurt from the top tray.

The house was warm and quiet, and I enjoyed the early morning light streaming through the blinds. My stomach demanded instant nutrition, so I quickly shoveled three heaping bites in my mouth. *Eat slow,* Mira had instructed me on the way home. *It fills you up faster and you eat less.* I sighed and forced myself to wait a minute in between bites.

Mom walked into the room, interrupting my thoughts on a pop quiz I expected that morning. Mom had always been lovely thanks to careful attention to skin care and a slender frame. After Dad passed, her once beautiful laugh lines disappeared into worried frowns. She wasn't slender anymore; she was downright skinny. *Too* skinny. She and

McKenzie were a page from the same book, while I received Dad's thick, big-boned frame. At least, that's what *he* always called it. I just figured I was chubby because I always had one hand in a box of cookies while the other rooted for our favorite baseball team from where we sat on the couch. Mom and Kenz bonded over shopping and walks around the block. Dad and I bonded over football games and hot wings.

Lots of hot wings.

"Good morning, Lexie," Mom said, with a measured note in her voice. Her eyes flickered to the yogurt in my hand, then back to my face in surprise. I could almost see her thoughts.

Yogurt? Is this Lexie eating light yogurt? Not the sugary, childish tube kinds?

"Hey, Mom," I replied. *Play it cool,* I thought. Mom knew I was going to the *Health and Happiness Society* with Bitsy, but we hadn't talked about it. Every time the words *calorie, diet,* and *scale* popped up in this house, a volcano threatened, and all of us eventually ended up spewing the lava of tears and anger. Typically Kenz took Mom's side in a lecture on my health, backing me into an emotional corner that I could only get out of by eating. The cereal in the cupboard called my name just thinking about it.

Mom slipped past me, grabbed a whole wheat muffin from the bread box, and a knife from the drawer.

"How was your morning?" she asked.

Translation: did you actually go to the gym and work out? Am I just seeing things?

"Good."

I finished the final scoop of yogurt with a sense of accomplishment. One healthy choice down. The container landed right in the garbage can and I reached for an orange in a bowl on the counter. Mom tensed, watching every movement from the corner of her eyes, seeming to wait for the moment I broke this healthy facade and grabbed a handful of those chocolate covered doughnuts with the yellow cake in the middle. They had—

I cleared my throat and shook my head, forcing my fingernails into the peel of the orange.

Bradley, I reminded myself. *Diet. Stick with it.*

The ugly truth loomed like a black cloud: just being in the same room as my mom made me want to eat. I'd been aware of it ever since she put me on a diet at ten. Mom worried about everything, and like a satellite, I picked up her anxiety and chewed my way through it like a Christmas ham. To be fair, it *had* been years since I'd shown any interest in losing weight, and then Dad had died, and I didn't care about anything.

Mom studied my clothes, which still had a ring of sweat around the armpits. Evidence. Rats. I'd have to change at the gym or shower before breakfast next time to avoid this heavy awkwardness.

"How was the gym?" she asked. If her words had been glass, they would have shattered from being so thin and delicate.

Translation: Do I have hope for an attractive daughter in the future?

She kept moving the same blob of peanut butter around the top of the already severed muffin. Creamy, of course, because Mom thought chunky had extra calories they didn't put on the label.

"Fine," I replied.

Mom and I hadn't *really* argued in a month, which meant we hadn't spoken either, not since Kenz came home from her date to announce her engagement to Casey, her dreamy fiancé that looked just like a Ken doll. They wanted to get married in the summer, and Mom immediately said, "That's perfect Kenz! It gives Lexie time to lose that weight and slim down for a bridesmaid dress."

Magma exploded from my livid mountain of rage, of course. We'd gotten into a yelling match, and all of us ended up in our separate rooms crying.

"I just want you to be happy and healthy and young again, Lexie!" Mom had said, her lower lip trembling. "You aren't happy. You're overweight. You're unhealthy. You're going to die just like your father and I can't lose anyone else! I just can't!"

Translation: You're not good enough, Lexie.

A stash of Little Debbie snacks in my closet downstairs started screaming at me. Fudge Rounds and Swiss Rolls. Classics. The frosting in the middle was the best part, obviously. The orange peel spritzed when I peeled it apart, sending a citrus tang into the air, reorienting me in the moment.

Little Debbie is not my friend. Little Debbie is not my friend.

Mom poured a small glass of grapefruit juice, set her muffin on a plate, grabbed a napkin, and arranged it all at the end of the table before she sat down for a first, careful bite. Everything perfect and in its place, as usual. She chewed every mouthful at least twenty-five times. *Helps digestion,* she always explained.

"Do you have any classes today?" she asked, her back to me now so I didn't see her probing eyes. I carefully split the orange in half.

"Yeah, Lit 402 and a biology class I have to take."

"Any homework?"

I turned to eye Mom in suspicion. She hadn't inquired about my classes or schoolwork in weeks. I couldn't deny it was nice to get her undivided attention at least once without Kenzie flittering around like a butterfly, distracting Mom with wedding plans and tulle colors.

"Pop quiz and a paper to turn in. Not too bad. I work this evening."

She nodded once, staring out the window in thought. I had a glimpse of her attractive profile bathed in the slatted sunlight shining in from outside, and felt sad. Her lips drooped in a perpetual frown. The skin that she'd taken such good care of was wrinkled now, and the light had vanished from her eyes. Dad had been gone for two years, but Mom still seemed weighed down by his absence. He certainly hadn't been perfect, and she had been hard on him, but she truly had loved him.

The orange had a surprisingly sweet flavor this morning—likely because it wasn't competing with the half cup of sugar that came with my usual cereal—so I sucked all the juice and enjoyed the taste as I ate in the silence. Once I finished, I tossed the peel in the garbage, grabbed my phone, and headed for the basement. I stopped at the door.

"Thanks for the chat, Mom," I said, glancing over my shoulder. She attempted a smile, something I hadn't seen from her in months. Feeling better, though still not ready to talk with Mom about my dieting plans, I headed downstairs with a happy heart and a smile of anticipation. The comfort of my morning ritual of stalking Bradley's Facebook page always made my day better.

Although, admittedly, this hadn't been a bad morning.

Chapter 9—Goth for the Day

A pile of textbooks slammed to the table, startling me from my lesson on formatting. My best friend Rachelle dropped into the chair across from me with a heavy thud.

"I need a brownie right now. I'm about to go Godzilla on all these poor innocent people if I don't get carbs in my belly."

I rolled my eyes. She had always enjoyed subtle entrances.

Today she wore her *Fairy of the Darkness* outfit, a veritable display of black. She must have been in the mood to *embrace the beauty of the night* again. Rachelle moved through fashion statements as fast as I could eat a plate of bacon. Today her eyeliner looked like it had been applied with a paint roller. Her bangs, cut in a straight line across her forehead, fluttered in a breeze blowing through the cafeteria. A small clump were dyed bright pink. No doubt with the washable hair dye she bought at the corner grocery store every now and then.

"Did you watch *Phantom of the Opera* again?" I asked. She sighed.

"I can't help myself. Every time I hear Gerard Butler sing "Music of the Night," I just want to slip into my inner goth, throw him to the ground, and make passionate love to him. I mean it's just not fair, right? No man should be that beautiful."

I laughed.

The smell of pizza and something fried wafted through the cafeteria, which was already a cacophony of smells and sounds. Rachelle and I always studied here. The noise and distraction helped me concentrate, and Rachelle liked to stay close to food. An argument I never disagreed with.

From the first day we met at eight years old when she had just moved into our town, our collective weight bonded us together. Because of Rachelle, I wasn't the only chubby kid on the playground. Most kids were too frightened of her to poke fun at us. When Jimmy Willgard called her fat in third grade, she gave him a wedgie so big he had to go home.

"Best suspension I ever had. Mom gave me a bowl of ice cream for sticking up for myself," she'd told me proudly. "Chubby kids have feelings too, you know? Why is it okay to make fun of *us?*"

From then on, she protected me, and I loved her. When Dad died, she remained after the funeral, Ben and Jerry's in one hand, Kleenex in the other. Unlike me, who tried to hide behind loose hoodies in shame, Rachelle embraced her weight, and, in some ways, loved to flaunt the fact that *she* could wear almost anything a skinny girl could wear.

That didn't mean it looked good, or wasn't embarrassing, but that wasn't the point to Rachelle.

"We need more fat people appreciation," she'd often say, fist raised in the air. "Down with *The Biggest Loser!* Down with the syndicates! Freedom for chubbies! Save Tibet!"

"Heard from Bradley?" she asked, smacking a wad of pink bubble-gum the same color as her pink highlight. She blew a bubble and it popped in her face. On cue, my phone flashed with a new text message from the handsome man himself. We'd been conversing during my literature class.

"Yeah," I said, grabbing the phone and slipping it into my pocket. I itched to answer him, but didn't want to with Rachelle around. Even though she was my best friend, I still didn't like her knowing about Bradley. I felt very protective of him—or maybe just the dreams I'd formed about him—and wanted to keep him wrapped in a cocoon. "How was class?"

She rolled her eyes. "So boring. But look what the English department just posted. I saw it on the ground when I strolled by and thought you might be interested. Sorry about the footprint."

She slapped a dirty piece of paper on the table in front of me. Bold words across the top declared: *Three Slots Available. Applications due June 15th.* Below that came the words that nearly stopped my breath: *Competitive Two-Month Publishing Internship with Delta Publishing in New York City. Available for all English, Communications and Creative Writing majors.*

"Rachelle!" I whispered in disbelief, "This is exactly what I want."

"Yeah. I know. I'm awesome." She blew another bubble but popped it on her own, then sucked it back into her mouth. "Hey, I brought money to buy us a pizza today. Mom's on a health kick again and moved all the good stuff out of the house, so I have to get my junk food kick here."

"Again?" I asked, still perusing the flyer.

"Yeah. She does it once a month, then realizes how tasteless romaine is, and goes back to what we know: pizza rolls and sausage sandwiches."

She stood up, her black tulle fairy skirt sticking out from her waist when she moved. Fishnet tights covered legs as chubby as mine. Rachelle had courage I would never have. I couldn't even wear yoga pants.

"I already ate," I said with a guilty smile, and her eyes dropped to the empty salad container next to me. I'd left class early to get here before Rachelle for this very purpose.

"Is that a salad?" she asked.

"Yeah."

She reared back as if I'd slapped her. Two pudgy hands rose in the air, decorated by a ring with a skull and an oversized fake ruby.

"Shut. The. Door. Since when do you eat *salad?*"

"It just sounded good."

"You aren't on a health food kick like my mom, are you?" Her black-as-night eyes narrowed on me in studious detail.

"It's just a salad, Rachelle."

"But it represents so much more," she retorted with a little pout. "You can't go be one of those snotty, skinny girls on me, you know. We're big girls, Lex. We always have been. It's who we are and who we'll always be. In some cultures, we'd be considered gods."

It's not who I always want to be.

I forced a smile to turn the conversation back to lighter topics. "You would, maybe. Just because having a tribe of aborigines worshipping you is probably on your bucket list."

"Obviously." She rolled her eyes, waddling away, tulle skirt bouncing. Her mutterings drifted away with her. "Salad? Like eating cardboard with olive oil on top, or something. Blech."

I let out a long, relieved breath, grateful the cat was out of the bag. Rachelle would be over it by the time she returned. I'd tell her about my diet . . . eventually. While she was gone, I quickly pulled up my calorie counting app to enter the details.

"Ranch?" I glanced at the serving size of the package that had come with the salad and my eyes popped out of my head. "I ate three hundred calories in just *ranch?*"

The addition of the chicken, the dried cranberries, the caramelized pecans, the blue cheese, and the bag of apple slices added up to a whopping number of calories I had not expected. I smacked my forehead with my hand. Weren't salads healthy? Did I get extra points for eating lettuce?

"This is not going to be as easy as I thought," I said with a sigh, tucking my phone back into my pocket. Thanks to a healthy breakfast, and avoiding the fun fruit packages I *used* to eat during classes, my diet today wasn't totally ruined. I'd have enough space for dinner.

Whatever rabbit food it would have to be.

Rachelle returned with a pizza and another dramatic entrance. It smelled like pepperoni heaven when she lifted the lid and waved it under my face.

"Dontcha want some?"

I grabbed onto my sanity before it ran away by breathing through my mouth to avoid the smell. Pizza sounded *divine.* Whoever had made this one had been extra generous with the cheese. Although my inner fat girl was throwing her fists against my stomach walls, demanding to be fed that luscious pile of cheese and grease, I pursed my lips and shook my head. If I ate a slice of pizza, I'd have to eat lettuce for dinner to stay on track.

"No, but thanks."

Rachelle's eyes lit up. "Wow," she said, grinning and snatching a slice. "Respect, Lex. I've never seen you turn down pizza."

I let out a sigh, surprised by how good it felt to refuse it.

"Thanks."

Chapter 10—Diet Dr Pepper

Except for the low drone of the TV in the background broadcasting an old baseball game, the pub remained silent and empty that night. Waking up early to exercise had thrown off my usual routine, so I enjoyed the near-quiet with a little sigh and another drink of my favorite medical personality, Diet Dr Pepper.

After defying all odds and refusing to have a slice of pizza with Rachelle at lunch, I went to my last class, then to work. Now my boss Pat stood behind the counter at the opposite end, head tilted back, thick, hairy arms hanging at his sides, gaping at the old TV hanging above the bar. He'd already seen that particular game twenty times, but still watched it with rapt attention.

With no customers around, my options for work dwindled significantly.

Homework? I thought. *Done.*

Glasses clean? I glanced at the dishwasher underneath the counter. *Running.*

Tables wiped? My nose wrinkled as I surveyed the tables in the room. Walking to each table didn't have a lot of appeal. *No, but that can wait until later. Like, the next shift.*

All my arithmetic meant there was nothing left to do until a customer showed up. A giddy rush swept through me. Time for my favorite pastime of all.

Eating.

I pranced to the back, regretting it when the muscles on top of my leg—whatever those were called—protested the movement. I'd expected to be sore immediately after working out, but it hadn't happened, so I'd fallen into false security. The soreness had started settling in like it meant to stay hours after the gym. The less I moved, the less it hurt, but the tighter it became. I had no idea how to get rid of it.

"Why do people exercise if it just hurts?" I asked no one, slowing to a walk. Food had never given me pain. I glanced down at my ample belly and grimaced. Well, not *physical* pain anyway.

The metallic fridge in the back of the pub was a beautiful sight to behold; two doors, a chrome-like exterior, and large enough to fit a couple of Lexies inside, which was saying something. I used to call it the magic portal to happiness. Instead of reaching for the handle and tugging it open, however, I stared at it. It wasn't really the magic portal to happiness, was it? No.

More like the magic portal to my next stop: 300 pounds.

Like a sick video that I couldn't get rid of, I replayed the moment when Bitsy weighed me in at 259 pounds. Although the rush of shame and disappointment still felt hot, I also remembered the euphoria of refusing the pizza that afternoon.

If I could refuse pizza with Rachelle, I could refuse dinner with Pat. There was nothing in that fridge that I'd be able to eat only 400 calories worth of and stop myself, and that's all I had left for the day.

"Fine!" I glared at the fridge. "I'll eat when I get home. I hope you're happy, magic portal of misery!"

My eyes drifted to a clock in the back with cats all over it. Pat had a sick fascination with the creatures, and owned at least twenty. One hour. I had one hour left to bide my time and stay away from the fridge of goodness.

With a dramatic turn, I marched out of the back and into the front. Still empty.

"What do I do?" I whispered in a panic. I wasn't used to passing my time without food in hand! If I didn't find something, I'd succumb, and with hunger like this, I'd eat *everything* in the fridge.

Bitsy's voice popped into my head like a mental drill sergeant, as if she could detect my cowardly thoughts from afar.

Even if you can't work out, just keep your body moving as much as you can.

Oh, great. Now I'd actually work instead of eating. Pat would likely send for an ambulance. Just to bolster myself in preparation, I drank another swig of DDP. Cold, icy goodness.

If I hadn't loved Bradley—or the idea of him—so much I would have taken my wedding vows out with DDP. No guilt, plenty of caffeine to keep me going, and tasted better than water. An arrangement I rather liked at the moment, when the magic portal kept taunting me to walk into lands of food and fun.

Logging DDP on my phone? Too easy! *Zero calories, suckers.*

I left Pat to continue silently reliving his glory days as a semi-pro baseball player and reached for a dishcloth. The tight muscles in my arms and upper back protested. This exercise thing was seriously overrated. With a wince, I wrung out a dishcloth and made a second round to wipe down already clean tables.

The mindless work of straightening chairs, tables, and sweeping loosened my tight muscles. Was that how it worked? The more I moved, the less sore I felt? Seemed liked a lot of extra work and movement.

I allowed my thoughts to drift to the day I would meet Bradley. I'd wear a black dress because . . . hello? Slenderizing. But it wouldn't matter because I'd already left the magic portal behind and would be skinny. As far as my hair, I was thinking of—

"I'm giving up Pepsi."

I leapt back, frightened out of my daydream by Mira's abrupt voice in my left ear. The fast move shoved my derriere right into the sharp corner of a table behind me, scattering a salt and pepper shaker. My hand flew to my chest.

"Good grief, Mira!" I cried. "Why did you scare me?"

She smirked. "Dreaming of Bradley?"

"No! O-of course not. I'm just . . . working."

She eyed the clean tables. "I can see that. I normally don't see you leave the bar unless you have to. What's the occasion?"

"I'm trying to move a bit more."

Moving around seemed like such an obvious thing, something most people did— but I didn't. Having to admit that I didn't even like doing simple tasks was embarrassing. Mira shrugged, and I realized again that I was in good company.

"Me too. That's why I walked here instead of driving."

Mira didn't live far away, maybe half a mile, but the thought of her walking surprised me. "Oh," I said. "On top of working out this morning?"

"Yeah."

I blinked several times. I'd never thought of working out *and* doing active things later. Didn't the morning trip to the gym cancel out the need to exercise later in the day? Did people actually exercise twice?

"I guess I never thought of that," I said lamely.

"Listen." She stabbed me in the chest with her finger. "I'm giving up pop and I think you should too. Will you do it with me?"

Her original statement wafted back through my mind. I blinked and stared at her in utter disbelief. Mira give up pop? She drank Pepsi like mother's milk, right up until she went to bed, caffeine and sugar notwithstanding. Her body had become so used to the brown serum that I assumed all her cellular processes depended on it.

"You're what?"

"Giving up Pepsi." She winced. "It's not going to be easy."

After regaining my composure and breathing again, I straightened the fallen salt and pepper shakers. My eyes darted to the sweating glass of DDP waiting for me on the bar, beckoning like a siren song. *Don't give me up,* it called. *Don't leave me!* Pat had turned his attention from the game and was glancing at Mira from the corner of his eyes every four or five seconds.

"I decided to do it after leaving the gym this morning, but I've already given in," she admitted. "I don't think it's something I can do on my own."

"Give in?"

"I normally drink a can with every meal, and in between, but I couldn't make it past lunch today!" She plopped her heavy bottom into a chair, her loose stomach and breasts moving like water under her muumuu. "To be honest, I'm not sure I *can* give it up. But Bitsy gave me some pamphlets on diabetes and how unhealthy pop is, and now I can't get it out of my head. What if I have to start taking insulin? What if my weight is just fat stores from all the sugar? What if—"

"Mira, Mira," I said, putting a hand on her shoulder. This kind of frantic talking had to stop. Giving up pop? Ludicrous. "Calm down. Why don't you just take it easy on the Pepsi? Instead of drinking three a day, just drink one over the whole day."

She grumbled something I couldn't hear.

"What?" I asked.

"I drink *five* a day."

"Oh. Well, make a goal to just drink two tomorrow."

She thought it over. "I suppose I could try."

I sat on the chair across from her. "If I can avoid the fridge here, you can cut down by three Pepsis."

"How did your day go?" she asked morosely. I sighed when my stomach grumbled.

"I hate it."

"Me too." She pressed her lips together. "I never realized how much I ate every day. I'm five hundred calories over my goal."

"I'm under," I said, "but totally miserable and starving and grumpy."

She smiled weakly and asked, "Think this will all be worth it?"

I imagined the black dress I wanted to wear when I met Bradley, how shiny and perfect my hair would look, and the lines of a skinny face I'd never seen before.

"I hope so," I said, pressing a hand to my aching stomach. "Because today has at least shown me that it's certainly not going to be fun."

Chapter 11—The Long Two Miles

Lexie, wake up.

The bright glow of Mira's text message shone on my face like the flashlight of a cop peering into my car. I groaned, rolled onto my stomach and squinted, mustering all my concentration into a response.

No.

Satisfied that I'd allayed the beast, I set the phone down and drifted back into the sweet, downy layers of sleep and rest. Not ten seconds later, my phone chimed with the happy chirp of a lark right in my ear. A lark I wanted to grab by the beak and throw across the room.

GET UP NOW! You know I'll come down there.

"Mira!" I growled, even though she couldn't hear me. "It's 5:30 in the morning! I don't have class on Fridays."

As if she'd heard me, another text came through.

I don't care how early it is, and I know you don't have class. Get out here. Now. I'm in your driveway waiting and I HAVEN'T HAD A PEPSI. We're going to the gym.

With a moan that would have impressed even my drama-mama sister, I shoved the covers off and fell out of bed with the *plop* of a baby whale dropping.

I hauled my still-asleep body off the floor and groped blindly for a pair of workout clothes. Except I didn't have "workout clothes" because I'd never worked out before yesterday in my life, so I grabbed a pair of loose sweats and another oversized shirt. After yanking my hair back into a ponytail, slipping on a pair of tennis shoes that needed replacing over a year ago, and fumbling my way through a hoodie, I tottered outside. Mira gave me a sweeter-than-sugar kind of smile when I fell into her car with less grace than a toddler learning to walk.

"See?" she asked with the menacing kind of tone that meant she was about to bite my head off. Mira without Pepsi was like a baby snake that couldn't control its venom. "Don't you already feel better?"

I shot her a blinding scowl, jerked the hoodie over my face, and sank into the seat with a phrase my mom wouldn't be proud of.

The gym was quiet except for the whir of machines and the questionable grunts coming from a guy near the weight rack. Mira hopped back onto an elliptical, bright blue leggings on and sweat band in place. Remembering my previous experience, however, I opted for the safety of the treadmill. To my supreme luck, I stood right below the TV with reruns of *The Golden Girls* playing. If I was going to be tortured, at least I could laugh my way through it. I set my pace at three miles per hour—which seemed pretty ambitious since I couldn't remember the last time I'd walked fifty feet when I wasn't forced—and started moving.

An episode and a half later, I glanced down in shock.

"What the crap? I just walked a mile and a half."

To say I was shocked I hadn't died is an understatement. A mile seemed so . . . long. And I'd done, not only one, but almost two. The excitement was so real I didn't know how to handle it, so I just kept walking. I looked back to the numbers, saw the maze of bright lights flashing, and figured I might as well finish off two miles.

Once *The Golden Girls* had finished, an old rerun of *Matlock* came on, so I turned my attention to people-watching again. The two girls lifting weights weren't there that morning, which disappointed me, but the Asian man running around the track had returned and puffed by every few minutes. The last half-mile finished interminably slow, and I was glad to step off the machine after forty minutes of constant walking.

That *had* to be a record for me. One of which I felt quite proud.

Elated, I found Mira standing stock still on the elliptical again, head angled back so far that her mouth tilted open, drooling over the news anchor for the local morning news.

"Hey!" I called across the running track. "Mira! I just walked two miles!"

She startled out of her reverie and automatically began moving her legs again. After a blink or two, she processed what I'd said and gave me a thumbs up.

My gaze travelled to the rest of the gym, where various people contorted themselves in painful positions to achieve something, I couldn't tell what. Should *I* try a new machine? One woman kept spreading her legs open and closed like a hussy. I shook my head.

No machines for me.

I couldn't even get off an elliptical without falling on my face. I'd surely kill myself on the weight machines. Or, I shuddered to think, get stuck in one and need help getting out. I imagined myself stopping a passerby.

Uh, excuse me? Could you find a spare forklift to heave my body out of this contraption? I'm stuck.

Seeing me frozen in deliberation, Mira climbed off her elliptical— successfully, I might add—with a heavy sigh.

"I'm beat," she said, wiping nonexistent sweat off her forehead. "Let's go. I just don't have a lot of energy this morning."

I cocked an eyebrow. "No Pepsi to get going?"

"No," she snapped. "Now stop talking about it. My body doesn't know how to function without it, okay? This dieting thing is just . . ." She trailed off, letting the words linger in the air unspoken.

I knew exactly what she meant.

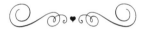

Once home, I slipped into my shower to wash off remnants from the gym. When the steam cleared from my mirror, I looked like a drowned rat clutching a towel because I couldn't wrap it around my body.

"That will be awesome," I thought, daydreaming of a time when I'd be able to wrap an entire towel—and not the oversized ones my mom bought just for me at Costco—all the way around my torso. I inspected my face and poked at the pudge of my neck with a finger, wishing I could target areas of my body to lose weight from first. *Zap!* There goes my double chin. *Pow!* There go my hamster cheeks.

How long did this weight loss thing take to happen anyway? Would I start seeing it come off in a day or two, or did it take months and months of slaving at the gym?

After changing into my usual baggy black pants and an old t-shirt of my dad's, I dropped back onto my computer chair to stare at the clock. Only 7:30 in the morning, and I felt wide awake. I normally slept in until eleven o'clock or noon on Fridays. Then Rachelle and I went out to Chipotle to get burrito babies.

What on earth was I going to do all day?

Duh! I thought with an eye roll. *Stalk Bradley.*

Unfortunately, Bradley wasn't online, so I satisfied myself with clicking through pictures of him until my stomach growled.

"What madness is this?" I asked, pressing a hand to my stomach. "You're hungry? Well of course you are! I didn't feed you much yesterday."

Visions of sausage, cheese, and egg sandwiches danced through my head, but Bitsy's stern face broke through them, and I sighed.

Egg whites for me, I supposed.

My eyes drifted to the calendar on my wall. I'd ended the day before exactly on target for my calories, which likely accounted for why I felt so ravenous today. I grabbed a sharpie and wrote a smiley face. It looked so nice that I wrote just beneath it:

Walked 2 miles.

With a sprightly spring in my step, I started for the stairs, wondering just how to separate the egg yolk from the white.

♥
Chapter 12—The Girl on TV
♠

It took me all of ten seconds after breakfast to find myself sitting in our front room, searching for the remote. With an egg white omelet sitting in my stomach—just barely satisfying the hungry, insatiable beast—I settled in for my favorite pastime.

Television.

With full time school and work part time, I didn't get a lot of bonding time with our TV anymore, and I missed the brainlessness of it. When I watched stories unfold, I forgot my own shame, my own grief, and if a box of sweet candy became involved, my depression. The taste of sugar overrode how much I really hated myself.

The memories of sitting with my dad, sharing a bowl of popcorn with extra butter while laughing at Seinfeld lived again when I resumed my usual place on the couch. Over time, the cushion had perfectly formed to my bottom. I sighed.

Feels so good.

It seemed kind of sad that I would mostly think of Dad while doing nothing except eating, but I pushed the thought aside. I flipped through the stations just to reorient myself to the channels. I'd never watched TV this early because I never woke up this early, except for class. Despite the early morning hour—it was just past eight, which still seemed an unholy time to be awake on a day off—there were still definite possibilities. An old rerun of *Friends* popped up, but of course it would be the Thanksgiving episode that showed Monica fat, so I flipped to a different station.

"Hey. What on earth are you doing awake right now?"

Our front door slammed open, and McKenzie strolled in like a Greek goddess just returning from her morning ablutions with the mortals. Her long hair, straight instead of frizzy like mine, hung in a ponytail down her back. She wore one of those cute workout outfits, the kind I'd be arrested for trying to wear, with the tight black leggings and form-fitting long sleeved shirt. Her face was flushed from the cold morning air, which meant she'd just returned from her daily run.

"Oh. I . . . I couldn't sleep."

She cast me a wary look, then gracefully lowered her ballerina body to the floor and contorted her legs into a stretch. I grabbed a pillow and hugged it to my stomach.

"You never wake up before eleven on a Friday," she said.

"Well today I did."

"Hmmm." Her eyes slipped to the TV, which had landed on a rerun of Jerry Springer. It promised to be one of the violent ones, so I left it there for the moment. Nothing made me feel better about my life than watching others who had screwed up theirs.

"So . . . nice run?" I asked, feeling pressed by the awkward silence to make conversation. When McKenzie wasn't nagging me about losing weight for her wedding, or spouting off sonnets about her Casey, the two of us didn't speak much. We had nothing in common. Kenz was too much like Mom: the living embodiment of everything I wasn't.

"Yeah, it was good," she said, frowning down at a massive computer-watch on her wrist. "I pushed myself and went six miles instead of the usual four, but I had to slow my pace to make it."

"Six?" I cried, my eyes bugging out of my head. The blood in my legs still seemed to be pumping from my two mile treadmill walk that morning. I couldn't imagine adding four more miles *at a run*. Some things in this universe were just not feasible, and getting my body to move at those speeds was one of them.

"Wow, Kenz. That's . . . that's great. Six miles would be really tough."

Her eyes narrowed on me from where she lay folded over her legs. I glanced away again. My stomach would never permit me to stretch that far. It would stop me like a plug in a bathtub. The sudden urge for a bag of Funyuns overcame me, so I hugged the pillow tighter.

"Sure," she drawled. "Great. Listen, Mom said that Mira—"

"I'm not doing anything with Mira!" I snapped, self-conscious that Kenz would know about my diet and workouts. This was *my* thing. I didn't want Kenzie butting in on it to label it as *sister bonding time* and try to join us at the gym. I'd look like the Stay Puft Marshmallow Man on a treadmill next to her.

Kenzie recoiled. "Calm down, I was just going to say that Mira agreed to do my wedding cake."

"Oh." I relaxed back against the couch. "Oh, that's great."

"It'll save me a lot of stress and money," Kenz said, redirecting her long, lithe legs into a pretzel stretch. "Heaven knows we're tight on money."

A current of stress came into her voice. Dad had some life insurance, but after all the medical bills, the funeral costs, and paying off some other debt Mom didn't speak about much, the remains wouldn't stretch very far. With both Kenzie and I going to school and living at home, Mom had gotten a job as a receptionist to help pad the empty slots.

And a wedding was a *big* empty slot.

"How are wedding plans?" I asked, flipping to another station. Jerry just wasn't doing it this morning. Nothing on TV seemed all that interesting now that the issues of my messed up family—or maybe just myself—found a spotlight.

"They're okay. Now that the dresses are picked out and ordered I'm not as stressed out."

I kept my gaze schooled away from her. I had no intention of wearing that pink horror of a bridesmaid dress to her wedding. None. The reminder of how puffy I'd looked forced me to push away the thought of how delicious a few maple flavored breakfast sausages would taste right then.

"Yeah, I'm sure that's a big stress off of you."

Kenzie stood up with the grace of a queen. How we were sisters, I'd never know.

"Yeah, let's hope."

She moved away before I could say anything else. The pit of self-pity that I fell into the moment she left was kind of pathetic. With a scowl, I flipped through the stations, deciding that I had all the calories left for the day that I wanted, so I deserved a snack.

I left the TV on an arbitrary station, having already made my mind up to cook a package of maple sausage links the way I'd been dreaming of—protein, right?—when I stopped halfway off the couch. The screen showed a popular weight loss TV show that Dad and I had watched once or twice, mostly while we were eating ice cream. We'd laughed about the idea of going to weight loss boot camp, trying to imagine ourselves on a treadmill or lifting weights.

It's not so bad, I surprised myself by thinking, remembering the triumph of my two miles. The taste of sausages would never compare to that feeling.

The girl that came on the TV screen next gave me pause. She looked just like me—depressed, overweight, and not unlike a tube sock stuffed with oranges. She stood on a scale, about to be weighed.

"Don't worry, sister," I murmured, hugging the pillow tight again. "I know *just* how terrible that feels. Except I didn't do it on public TV."

She buried her face in her hands when the numbers popped up on the scale. 262.

I gasped. She cried. I forgot all about breakfast sausages and sank back into the couch, my eyes riveted on the screen.

This girl was just like me.

I didn't really know how the show worked, I made it a point to avoid TV that involved exercise in any form, even if I wasn't supposed to participate, but it didn't matter. I *had* to see what happened next, because this girl was me, and I was her, and suddenly I didn't feel quite so alone, or stuck, in my big pit of pity.

The episode ended an hour later, shuffling onto a cheesy soap opera I couldn't stand. I peeled myself away from the television, found a bottle in the cupboard, filled it with ice water, and grabbed my keys. I was going to find out what happened to that girl.

Even if I had to buy every season of the show.

I left the house, and headed for Best Buy, unaware that I had totally forgotten to grab a snack before leaving.

Chapter 13—Frankenstein

Thanks to the hearty drama provided by reality TV reruns in DVD form, my day off slipped by in a surprising blur.

I shucked my usual date to Chipotle with Rachelle in favor of a yogurt container and another episode of watching other people sweat like pigs. Keeping my insatiable appetite reined in seemed easier when I saw results from other people. Their weight loss transformations made my eyes bug out.

If they did it, I could do it.

"What?" Mira asked Monday morning when I climbed into her car and waited for her to drive to the gym. "You're not going to snap at me? You're not going to get angry? Not even a glare?"

I glanced over in surprise. "About what, Mira?"

"Working out."

Her lips, which had an unnatural amount of bright lipstick for so early in the morning, were pressed into a bundle of hot pink disapproval.

"No. Why would I get angry?"

"Because you hate the gym. You hate early mornings. And you hate exercise. At least, you have the past couple of days."

Well, she certainly wasn't wrong. I still had a pit in my stomach just thinking about exercising around other people, my less-than-svelte frame perched on a machine that could buck me off at any moment, sending me to the ground in a fluid pile of fat and bones. My mind reviewed the TV episodes I'd been glued to, recalling the personal trainers yelling at the contestants, motivating them to lose weight and be healthier people, and I shook my head.

"I'm not exactly excited about working out so early, but I'm not angry either."

Mira studied me like an alien life form, her eyes tapered, hands clenched on the steering wheel, one eyebrow ticked up. She must have decided I wasn't a hostile invader because she backed out of the driveway without another word.

"I went over my calories yesterday," she said once we parked in the gym lot, looking as forlorn and lost as a child. My seat belt snaked across my belly with a hiss. I stared at her.

"That's okay. I'm sure we'll all have less-than-perfect days."

Mira just sighed. "Yes. I suppose."

I put my hand on the doorknob, mimicking her sigh. *Here we go again.* "Let's get this over with, Mira."

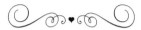

Hey! I didn't get a chance to talk to you all weekend. Seemed weird, didn't it?

Bradley's message popped up while I sat in my computer chair, printing off the homework I'd been ignoring all weekend. My printer chugged away, spewing pieces of paper onto the floor. Steam from my bathroom still curled into the bedroom from my shower after the gym, and I dreamed of a Jimmy Dean sausage sandwich that I wouldn't let myself eat because Bitsy's drill sergeant voice rang in my head.

Yes! I typed, wondering if I should have left the exclamation mark off. *I was pretty busy hanging out with some friends. How about you?*

I cocked my head to the side, nearly breaking my towel turban, and wondered if all the contestants on the TV show could be qualified as "friends." I sent it with a shrug. He'd never know.

Homework mostly for me this weekend, he replied. *Hanging out at my dinky apartment by myself, trying not to feel like a loser while my friends make their way across Europe.*

My heart clenched. His friends were in Europe? How wonderful would that be!

Oh? I returned, my heart hammering. *Where in Europe?*

Everywhere. Sounds like a blast, huh? I would have gone but I had to stay for school and practice.

I swallowed a little lump in my throat. Dad and I had always talked about travelling. Talked, mostly, because we didn't really do much. But he'd always wanted to see Spain, and I'd always wanted to see the

British Isles, so we'd agreed to do a week in each place. Then he'd died, and I hadn't really gone anywhere.

At all.

I hope you get to go one day, I replied quickly, lest he think I'd forgotten him while I fell into reveries. *Sounds great.*

How about you? You're so motivated to be an editor, you must have something going on this weekend, right?

"Right," I snorted. "The only thing I have going on is watching *other* people lose weight and live their lives while I try to figure out how to open a package of Donettes."

Donettes. *Mmmm.* Powdered sugar wrapped around a sweet, light pastry that—

Didn't you say something about an internship a few days ago? Bradley asked, jerking me from my daydream. *Sounds like that could really put you on the trajectory toward the editing career you've always wanted.*

My eyes fell to the flyer advertising the new internship that Rachelle had found. I'd tacked it on the corkboard behind my desk, where it stared at me every day. My eyes narrowed on it.

Three Slots Available. Applications Due April 15th.

Competitive Two-Month Publishing Internship with Delta Publishing in New York City. Available for all English, Communications, and Creative Writing majors.

Since winter still raged outside, I had time to ramp up my resume a little bit. If anything had motivated me in life, my career was it. I didn't want to be a writer, necessarily. I wanted to help other people find their words, perfect them, hone them, and release them into the world. The idea of being a cog behind the wheel appealed more to me than being visible, where people could critique and judge me. I resolved to speak with my advisor that afternoon and ask what I could do to get that internship.

Perhaps I wasn't totally lost.

Yet.

Yeah, I typed. *I'm actually speaking with my advisor about it this after-noon so I can give myself the best chance to win it.*

Awesome. Keep me updated on how it goes. Hey, I actually had a great idea the other day. Since you love to read, and I want to love to read (but I don't necessarily, I'd rather play sports) what if we both read the same book and then discuss it? I think I'd do more reading if something actually came from it afterward. I notice all the Goodreads reviews you do on Facebook and thought you might enjoy it.

I stared, unblinking, at his words. Was he serious? Did college guys *read* outside of textbooks and swimsuit magazines?

Uh, that sounds amazing, I replied, grateful he couldn't see the drool forming at my lips.

LOL. I don't really read for fun, so this will force me to take more time for it. It's a double bonus knowing you won't make fun of me for it. But let's read something cool, right? None of this romance, Jane Austen kind of stuff.

Obviously not.

I do have a tough guy image to maintain. :)

"Yeah," I agreed, pulling my towel turban off and letting my drying hair fall onto my shoulders. "The image of a perfect man."

How about we start with Mary Shelley's Frankenstein? I suggested. *She started writing it at eighteen. It does have a little romance in it, but it's mostly a gothic thriller. Stellar writing. You can't get better than the line "It was on a dreary night of November that I beheld the accomplishment of my trials."*

He started typing, then stopped. I waited with bated breath, berating myself.

"Stupid suggestion." I ducked my head into my hands. "I should have suggested something more manly like *All Quiet on the Western Front!*"

Sounds perfect, he said with the little chime of the chat notification. *I'll stop by the library today. Let's say we'll report back in two weeks for our online book chat?*

I released all the air from my chest in one great *whoosh.*

On my calendar.

Perfect. TTYL.

I stared at the computer screen with a happy, crooked smile. Discussion of a book. How wonderful. I hopped up from my computer chair, walked past my secret stash of Mallowbars tucked deep in the closet that called to me—what could further my joy except eating?—and into my bathroom.

I had an advisor to speak to.

Chapter 14—Doomsday #2

Wednesday approached a little like death—without warning.

I woke up that morning with no enthusiasm. Not even the thought of talking to Bradley on Facebook cheered me. Knowing I would have to face Bitsy in the evening for our weekly *Health and Happiness Society* meeting made a rock sink into my stomach and stay there all day.

I didn't necessarily fear Bitsy. I feared the scale.

After a week of sheer torture, what felt like major food deprivation, and constant calorie counting, I'd barely remained under my allotted number of calories each day. The fact that I'd made it to the gym six times felt heroic. I deserved a Macy's Parade float.

Never mind that I felt like I could be one.

While I felt proud of my restraint, I couldn't really enjoy it because I kept having nightmares that I'd step on the scale, and it would say *275*. Logically, there was no way I could have gained that much weight after taking away the daily Ho Ho's, but that didn't matter. My heart braced for the inevitable diet disappointment. I *knew* I would gain, and I'd realize how hopeless this entire endeavor was, and I'd fall face first into a molten lava cake.

"Welcome back!" Bitsy chirped from the top of her living room that evening. A few squeaks sounded from the back rooms, sounding like the shrill cry of girls playing together, and not very nicely at that. Bitsy wore a baggy shirt, workout pants, and a pair of old sneakers with holes in the side. Although she'd put on plenty of makeup, her skin had a moist sheen to it, as if she'd just finished working out. Her collection of exercise DVD's seemed taller than last week, and I wondered if I'd have enough discipline to turn off the TV and actually work out at home.

Doubtful. Mira still had to drag me out of bed to go to the gym.

"Well, that's not much enthusiasm," Bitsy said with a frown, propping her hands on her hips like a scolding mother. In a sense, she was our weight-loss-Mama. "Aren't you guys excited about getting happy and healthy?"

"Praise the lawd!" Mira called, one hand in the air. The two men sitting on folding chairs across from Mira and me managed half-smiles. Bitsy pressed her gaze right into my eyes like she wanted to share her vision with me. Unfortunately, I had no desire to view myself from her eyes.

"Lexie?" she asked.

"Yes?"

"Are you excited about getting healthy?"

I'm excited about looking hot for Bradley.

"Yes, Bitsy," I said, feeling like a preschooler under duress. I couldn't even meet her eyes! Why didn't the military recruit her? She smiled, but her narrowed gaze suggested that I still hadn't fooled her. She knew I was doing this for shallow reasons. But at least they were motivating shallow reasons.

"Wonderful," she replied, although her voice had a current of disappointment in it. "Well, let's get started, I suppose. We'll do the weigh-ins, talk about our week, and then I want to discuss the importance of drinking water, as well as a few food hacks to cut down calories but keep that delicious flavor!"

I ignored the urge to grab Bitsy's decorative pillow and hug it to my stomach, feeling suddenly insecure. That bloody scale awaited. I could feel it calling to me. Mira hopped up.

"I'll go first!" she called, waddling into the back behind Bitsy. She returned a few minutes later, face flushed and lips forming a straight line. I couldn't read her expression, so when Bitsy called one of the men back, I sent Mira a questioning glance. She shook her head.

"Bitsy said we're not supposed to share our results with each other."

"Seriously?"

Mira nodded, and I knew that I'd never find out. She viewed Bitsy as some sort of god. I rolled my eyes and stared at the carpet, wondering what Bradley was doing right then.

"Lexie?"

Bitsy's voice pulled me from my reveries of what Bradley would look like when we met. She flapped her hand at me.

"Let's go. You're the last one!"

My stomach clenched as I shuffled behind her and into the suffo-cating bathroom. The scale sat in the middle of the floor, an innocent enough contraption that didn't even know it was a device of torture and pain. How oblivious we all were to our own purposes in life.

Bitsy smirked. "You didn't wear a hoodie this time."

"Nope." I slid out of my flip-flops. "Or sneakers."

Ha! Take that! I've already started figuring out how to beat this scale!

I stepped on, and the chrome exterior felt cool under my bare feet. The numbers flipped and changed, whirring higher and higher until they suddenly stopped. My heart nearly beat out of my chest. I sucked in a deep breath, certain I was dreaming.

254

"Well," Bitsy said with surprise. "It looks like you've lost five pounds this week. That's equivalent to a two liter bottle of pop."

I put a hand against the wall to steady myself. Five pounds. I'd just lost two liters of root beer. Me, Lexie Greene, had lost five pounds for the first time in my life. This self-proclaimed junk food connoisseur and TV show hoarder had done the impossible.

"Wow. I thought I would gain."

"You didn't."

"I've never lost before. At least, not that I've tracked."

"Never? This is the first time you've tried to lose weight?"

"Yeah." I shrugged. "Dad and I just always ate and watched TV together. He made it seem like my weight wasn't really that impor-tant." Talking about my dad to Bitsy's steely expression wasn't easy, so I quickly changed the subject before she could ask further questions. "Will I be able to keep this going? I'm afraid that the weight loss is going to stop here."

Bitsy snorted. "Did you stick to the calorie allotment?"

Like a slave.

I nodded. "All week. Mira and I worked out together every day, except Sunday, too."

"Good. That's what you need to do. Now just keep at it. You might have a plateau or a stall or something, but you should be good to go."

"You make it sound so easy."

"It's not," she said, and a sudden haunted look came into her eyes. It disappeared as quickly as it came, but it made me wonder what lurked beneath the drill sergeant exterior. "But it's possible. Let's go. The others are going to wonder what kept us."

Like Mira, I schooled my expression into indifference, but secretly threw a party inside with glitter, lollipops, and lots of fluffy cupcakes. Five pounds! I needed a piece of cake to celebrate! Wait, no. That was counterproductive. I silenced the inner fat kid demanding that I acknowledge my accomplishment by eating, and instead accepted the bottle of water that Bitsy handed around.

Lame, I thought. *I've earned an éclair at least.*

"Water," Bitsy began, looking more comfortable now that she was in charge again, "is essential to all our bodily functions. . ."

Her voice trailed into the background. I actually listened this time, unlike the previous week. Seeing that results actually came from so much exhaustive work and deprivation had changed the game. Dreams of Danish pastries still danced in my head, so I drank the bottle of water as fast as I could. It made me feel sick, but at least my stomach was full.

"That's all I have today," Bitsy concluded twenty minutes later, after Mira finished a play-by-play of her daily calories. "Just remember that the second week is the hardest. If you had a big loss this week, you may not have a big loss next week. It's impossible to tell what our bodies are going to do, and some of us are still getting to know ourselves"

Her eyes fell on me. I knew my body just fine! And right now, it wanted Arby's curly fries stacked on a roast beef sandwich with two packets of fry sauce.

"Your challenge this week is to try three healthy new recipes, and bring them next week to share. I'll see you on Wednesday. Good work, everybody."

Chapter 15—No Freebies

"Thanks a lot, jerk!" I yelled, barely restraining the passive aggressive impulse to lay on the horn when a car cut me off. "You just made my day a lot more peachy!"

Settling for annoyed ranting instead of flipping the bird, I slowed down and forced myself to take a deep breath. To say it had been a long day would have given the misery no justice. The high of losing five pounds during the second *Health and Happiness Society* meeting the night before faded as soon as I woke up an hour and a half late. Mira had gone to the gym without me—although she still sent eight very angry text messages summarized in the words: *Don't fall off the bandwagon now that you've lost weight!*

I had scrambled as fast as I could, but still showed up late to my first class with my shirt on backwards. My eyes flipped to the papers I'd hurled onto the passenger seat, first catching the big red *D* scrawled across the top. The words *inability to meet objectives* came beneath.

"My worst grade ever," I whispered, shaking my head. I'd never scored below a *C* on a test in my life! Not even when I took Statistics, the most unholy course in all of humankind. My stomach growled in blatant reminder that it hadn't been fed it because I had to skip breakfast. I'd forgotten my wallet at home, and Rachelle didn't have class today, so I couldn't even raid a vending machine or borrow money.

The sign for Donut World popped into my line of vision on the road ahead. My eyes glazed over and I sucked in a deep breath. *What aches doesn't a cream-filled doughnut heal?*

None. Except maybe obesity, but in my frantic mind, I didn't care.

"Yep," I said. "This is going to happen."

The tires of my car squealed when I hooked a hard right and turned into the parking lot. Pushing aside my sense of self-pride with deliberate force, I dove into the nooks and crannies of my car, fishing for old change. Desperate for sugar, for the amnesia of emotions it always gave, I rooted around until I found a dollar in crusty change and threw myself inside the store. My food conscience silenced easier than I thought.

"It's just one doughnut," I told myself, standing in line behind a woman with a bright blue bouffant. "Just one. This won't kill the diet. Besides, I didn't eat lunch . . . or breakfast. This will be lunch. And breakfast. Besides, I just lost five pounds. I've earned this doughnut. I won't gain five pounds from a doughnut."

The strings of rationalizations ran through my head until I stepped to the counter. My eyes fell on a sign illuminated from holy light streaming from the heavens. Or a flickering fluorescent bulb just above, but whatever.

Two for One.

So the universe didn't really hate me today.

I slammed my money on the counter. "Two chocolate cream-filled. Make sure they're really filled, you know?"

The guy behind the counter gazed at me with an expression that said he recognized not only me—this certainly wasn't my first time coming here after a bad day—but the look in my eyes. He nodded.

"Got it," he said in a voice filled with understanding. With a tissue paper, he carefully selected the two most plump, shining doughnuts in the case. My mouth watered.

"Keep the change," I said when he handed me the brown bag, already spotting on the bottom from grease, and flew out of the store without another word. Relieved to get the sugary sweetness in my body, and more relieved to forget my bad day, I climbed in the car, turned up the radio to drown out my inner Bitsy, and bit into the first doughnut.

Forgetting my health came naturally once I tasted the sweet, sweet chocolate. I melted into the pastry, relieved to find happiness *somewhere*.

Despite, or because of, my hunger, I didn't really take the time to enjoy them. Before I'd even finished the first doughnut, I had the second in hand. Then they were gone, and I glanced in the bag, hopeful the employee had done me a solid by giving me a freebie.

No such luck.

Disappointed, and still hungry, I leaned back in my chair, licking the final remnants of chocolate off my face. Before I knew it, the buzz of tasting sugar began to fade.

"Dang," I muttered. Normally the euphoria of eating lasted longer. My phone buzzed, but I ignored it. Now that my stomach had tasted food again, it demanded more. Sighing, I started my car again and headed home, annoyed that food hadn't made the day better like it used to. No matter how I tried, all I could see as I drove were numbers.

259

At least it was just two doughnuts, I thought, but felt no comfort.

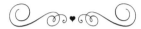

Mom's hysterical voice greeted me the moment I walked inside. I groaned and mentally prepared myself for her onslaught of emotions by dropping my bag of heavy books to the floor.

"Why didn't you answer your phone, Lexie? I've called twice. Where were you! You're normally home before this! Did you pick up my dry cleaning? I left you three messages."

"Sorry, Mom. It was a bad day."

"Why do you have a phone if you never pay attention to it?" she groused, and I found her in the kitchen, her face flushed and hair flying everywhere. "I needed you to pick up my dry cleaning!"

Just seeing my mom made my appetite increase. *Pizza rolls. Chicken nuggets. Lots of ketchup.* I stuffed the doughnut bag in the garbage and moved past her toward the fridge. *String cheese. Sugary yogurt. Corn dogs.*

"I'll go get it later," I said. "Let me get something to eat. It's been a long day."

"You're not the only one with a bad day!" she cried, picking odd pieces of trash off the counter. She hobbled around wearing only one shoe. "McKenzie got in a fight with her fiancé and took my car without asking, leaving me stranded. She's not answering her phone either, by the way! I had to call in sick to work, I've a ladies' gardening party that I'm running tonight, and I needed that dress so I could look presentable conducting! Now I'll be late for my own meeting."

Bagel bites. Bagels with cream cheese. Cream cheese frosting on a cinnamon roll.

Like McKenzie, Mom had never been good at dealing with stress. Her emotional anxiety was one of the reasons I gained more than fifty pounds after Dad died; supporting her and listening to her cry about how much she missed him had driven me right into the cold, constant arms of the fridge.

"Sounds like you should be angry at Kenzie, Mom," I said, grabbing the pizza rolls from the freezer, stuffing aside the nagging voice in my head that kept squeaking, *calories! Calories!*

Screw calories, I responded. *I've already eaten two doughnuts and missed the workout anyway. Might as well fall hard if I'm going to fall off.*

"Are you off your diet now?" Mom asked, aghast. She stood in front of the garbage, clutching her chest like I'd given her physical pain. "Doughnuts and pizza rolls?"

I closed my eyes. Mira must have been updating Mom on my life, because I hadn't said a word to her about my diet for just this purpose.

"No, I'm not off it. I've just had a bad day."

"Lexie! You can't expect to be thin if you turn to food the moment you have a bad day! You'll just binge eat the way you always do."

Better that I turn to food than take it out on my daughter, I thought, but kept silent, as I always had, and wished Dad were here to talk Mom down. Instead of responding, I arranged the pizza rolls in a circle on the outside of the plate, then snatched the leftover mozzarella sticks from the freezer and set them in the middle. Dad had taught me that arrangement to keep the cheese from melting out of the mozza sticks.

"So you're just going to ignore me?" Mom asked, throwing her hands in the air. "Just like your father used to do. You're just like him, you know! You don't care about me, or yourself, so you're just going to eat yourself into an early grave like he did. He left me know you know, and I blame him."

I winced. It wasn't the first time I'd heard the words, but they stung fresh every time.

"Oh, he didn't divorce me or anything," Mom continued, still waving her hands, moving around the kitchen with no purpose. "But he ate himself to death so he might as well have!"

Her voice ended on a sob, and she whirled around and stormed from the room, a can opener in hand. The tirade ended with the slam of her bedroom door.

My thoughts whirred as I stared at the rotating plate in the microwave. *Dad's gone. Mom's lost it. McKenzie had a fight with her fiancé. Failure to meet objectives. No lunch. Two doughnuts. Missed workout. Off the bandwagon. Mom blames Dad. So sad. Want to cry.*

As soon as my food finished, I grabbed a bottle of ranch, the last of the Ben and Jerry's, and headed into the darkness of my lair downstairs to forget all my problems in the sweet taste of carbs.

♥
....

Chapter 16—Better

....
♠

Within twenty minutes, the carnage of my eating binge had ended.

A ketchup-and-ranch-streaked plate sat empty in front of me, topped by an empty Ben and Jerry's container with a spoon sticking out the side. I stared at it with a blend of emotions.

"Oh no," I whispered. "I just ruined everything."

I dropped my face into my hands. The high of eating quickly subsided, just as it had with the doughnuts, and I sat in the aftermath with nothing left to think about but the shame of giving up. The numbers *249* flashed across my eyes. Surely, next week, they'd be even higher. I'd just doomed myself to an eternity of cyclical dieting and unending calorie counting.

"I'll never meet Bradley. I'll look like a bloated flamingo in the stupid bridesmaid dress and live in McKenzie's pictures forever."

Tears welled up in my eyes. Why did I do this? Why did I sabotage myself?

Just when my heavy thoughts of despair had turned to the Ho Ho's in the closet—despite my self-loathing for everything else I'd just eaten—my phone buzzed. Mira's number flashed across the screen, but I ignored it. It went to voicemail, and seconds later a text message came through.

I had a bad day. Let's go to the gym.

My eyes slipped to the clock above my desk. Almost seven o'clock. The gym? My forehead furrowed. I'd never heard of such a strange idea in my life. Who went to the gym at this time of day? Against my inner instinct to raid the fridge and wallow a bit more, I texted her back.

Uh, okay. I'll be ready in five.

I'm already in your driveway, so hurry up.

Although I didn't really want to go, escaping my self-imposed torture and prison sounded much better. If I stayed, I knew I'd just eat the Ho Ho's and further my downward spiral of shame. There had been plenty of nights in the past when the eating never stopped. At least I could cut it off somewhere tonight.

When I sat in the passenger seat, Mira was staring straight ahead, her hands at ten and two on the steering wheel.

"Hi," she said.

"Hi."

"I had an awful day," she whispered. "I drank six cans of Pepsi and only worked out this morning for twenty minutes without you there to motivate me to keep going."

I laughed in bitter irony, but tears had resurfaced again, so it came out as more of a wet chuckle. "I ate two doughnuts, half a plate of mozzarella sticks, half a pint of Ben and Jerry's and half a plate of pizza rolls because of *my* bad day."

"At least you only ate half of all those things," she pointed out. I snorted.

Mira looked over at me with a heavy sigh. "I thought losing weight would have made me more motivated to keep going, but it's like today I lost all my desire to keep up this new routine."

"Me too."

"It's so new, and so strange. I-I don't know how to . . . I don't know how to deal with my life without finding comfort in food, so in some ways it feels like everything is more difficult because I can't forget it by eating spaghetti." Mira dropped her head back against the seat rest. "This sucks."

I felt as if she'd taken the words from my very heart, and hearing them stated by someone else left me a little empty inside. *Wow,* I thought. *We are certainly messed up.* But at least if I was messed up, I wasn't alone.

"Me either," I admitted. "I got my worst test score ever, and I didn't eat lunch. It was a horrible day to start out, and then Mom and I got into a fight."

"I know. She called me and told me you were binge eating, but I was actually already thinking of begging you to go to the gym with me."

I pressed my lips together in silent fury. "Of course she did," I muttered, looking away.

I couldn't tell Mira how I *really* felt about how my mom's affection and approval depended on physical perfection. Hadn't she always been hard on Dad because he was overweight? Hadn't beautiful, skinny McKenzie been the favorite because she managed to stay trim and healthy?

"She loves you, you know," Mira said quietly. "I know it doesn't seem like it because she has a weird way of showing it, but losing your dad took almost everything out of her. She's terrified that she's going to lose you one day too. Trying to get you to lose weight makes her feel like she controls the situation more, so you won't die on her suddenly too."

My stomach rumbled even though I wasn't hungry, conjuring up images of a stack of banana pancakes, but I shoved it away. Energy this hot needed a *real* outlet.

"Let's go to the gym," I suggested, wiping a tear off my cheek. "I need to hit something."

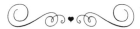

I walked on the treadmill first, but instead of keeping a slower pace so I could see the TV screen without bobbing up and down, I cranked the speed up to 3.8. My legs swished back and forth so fast that I nearly fell off twice, but after a minute or two of dogged determination, I found a stride, so to speak, and stuck with it through the evening news.

When a commercial popped up, my eyes strayed around the gym, finally landing on the two girls that I'd seen the first time I went to the gym. They worked around a set of weights in moves I didn't understand. Instead of feeling intimidated, I felt an odd kinship. Instead of binge eating pastries and Diet Dr Pepper, I was at the gym doing something just like those girls. The thought empowered me.

Friends popped up on TV next, and it felt so good to not be stuck at home in my usual mire of self-pity that I did something I'd never done before.

I jogged.

The guy on the treadmill next to me—whom I kept trying to ignore—ran like a gazelle at 7.0. I wanted to tell him to stop showing off, but spared the breath. Instead of walking at 3.8, I started a slow jog at 4.4 miles per hour.

I made it only thirty seconds before my side started to cramp, my breath came in awkward gasps, and I felt like dying, so I slowed back down to 3.4. I'd strategically chosen that particular treadmill because it had no mirrors by it, so I couldn't see if my fat rolls flabbed up and down in undulating waves with every step I took. To be honest, I didn't care. I just wanted to be a different Lexie today. I didn't want to be the one filled with self-loathing and shame.

So after I caught my breath, I increased the speed back to 4.4 again. This unusual pattern of walking/jogging persisted through the current episode of *Friends* and into the next. When my knees became wobbly and I felt as if I was going to throw up, I settled for a brisk walk. Mira toddled over.

"You ran," she whispered, eyes wide. "I'm impressed. Way to turn the day around!"

My hands clutched the top of the treadmill to keep from falling off. I moved my towel off the screen where it had hidden my numbers.

"An hour," I said in shock. "I've been doing this for an hour."

"Burned four hundred calories," she pointed out. "I think that's a decent counter to a bad day, don't you? Doesn't make up for it, of course, but I bet you feel better."

I stopped the treadmill, grateful to give my shaking legs a rest. If I put the thirty second time spans of running together, it wouldn't quite equal ten minutes. I'd mostly walked, but that didn't matter. I felt better. Loads better. The anger at my mom didn't consume me with the thoughts of food now. Although I still felt ashamed about my binge, I realized in hindsight it could have been worse. If Mira hadn't showed up, it *would* have been worse. Perhaps I hadn't totally lost the momentum of my diet.

"Yeah," I said with a lopsided smile. "I do feel better."

She returned my smile. "Come on, kid. Let's go. I'll buy you a bottle of water, my treat. We need to flush all this junk food out of our body now and start fresh again."

Chapter 17—People-Eater

"Why is bubblegum pink? Seems like a strange color, right? Why not purple? Or orange? What's up with pink anyway?"

Rachelle asked her stream of questions the next day while smacking loudly next to my ear, popping bubbles every ten seconds with her obnoxious wad of gum that looked suspiciously close to the shade of pink my sister wanted me wear as her bridesmaid.

"To annoy you," I responded. "Can you give me some breathing room?"

Rachelle sat almost on top of my lap in the cafeteria the morning after my shameful eating binge. She wore a Rainbow Brite Halloween outfit that she'd found at a plus size costume store two years before. She'd donned a bright blue top, a matching skirt trimmed with white fur that was *far* too short for anyone our size, and pulled her hair into a high ponytail with a piece of rainbow ribbon. Extremely bright rainbow tube socks went halfway up her calves, but couldn't make it any farther, so they'd rolled down to two different lengths.

"Sorreee," she sang as she scooted over, eyes narrowed on the other side of the room. "See that guy over there? The one that looks like he's wearing a toupee? I want to ask him on a date. He looks like he could eat a lot, then I wouldn't have to worry about holding back and would get free food. I'd probably make out with him, too."

She motioned to a group of IT nerds on computers, with headphones and microphones, submersed in a video game world. I couldn't imagine playing video games in a college cafeteria. But then, I never used to be able to picture a time in my life when I'd willingly diet, so the universe played all kinds of tricks on people.

"Go for it," I said, adding in a mumble, "in fact, do it right now so I can get this done."

Smack. Pop. Pop-pop-pop-pop-POP!

"Rachelle, cut the symphony, will you?"

She scowled. "What's got up your butt today? Is it because you're still eating rabbit food? You need a good dose of Little Debbie medicine."

I popped the mental visions of Fudge Rounds that danced in my head. "It has nothing to do with my salad," I muttered. Rachelle lifted an eyebrow, clearly detecting my blatant lie. I'd bought a salad for lunch again, only this time I opted out of the Ranch dressing and found a balsamic vinaigrette instead. "Vinegar speeds up your metabolism," Mira had told me the night before as she drove me home. "I'm going to start taking a shot of it every morning."

The thought made me want to hurl. Eating it in a salad hurt enough.

"Look," I said with an exaggerated sigh. "I'm trying to go through this registration before my next class. My advisor Miss Bliss gave me a few online classes I could take to beef up my resume for that internship, remember? I have to do it now because I work tonight."

"I remember. I gave it to you and by doing so practically saved your life," she retorted. "And yet there's still no gratitude."

"I said thank you."

"Nothing says thank you like sharing a Root Beer Float with me."

"I already told you, I'm not going to—"

"Ah ha!" she screamed, lifting a finger into the air and drawing the perturbed gaze of a cafeteria worker our direction. "You *are* on a diet, aren't you? Traitor to the big girls club! TRAITOR!"

I grabbed Rachelle's flailing hands and forced them back to her side. Thankfully, the ringing of my phone saved me out of a forced confession, so I recklessly answered it without looking at who called. "Hello?"

"Hey, is this Lexie Greene?"

I pressed a finger to my other ear and turned away from a chorus of *whoops* from the gamers on the other side of the room. "Yeah," I said. "This is Lexie. Who is this?"

"This is Bradley."

My stomach turned so cold that it spread through my body in a tingle as fast as lightning. The sounds of the cafeteria faded away. I stared at the lime green tile floor, eyes wide, mouth open, the blood draining from my face and pooling at my feet.

Dear heavens, I thought. *Bradley sounds as sexy as he looks on Facebook.*

"Hey, you there? Lexie? Lexie?"

"Uh, yeah, I mean yes. I-I'm here. How . . . how are you?"

I glanced discreetly to Rachelle. Luckily her gaze had narrowed back on the boy at the other side of the room with a patch of acne on top of his nose. She had the intent look of a hunter on her face and would attack in mere moments, no doubt.

"I'm great. So sorry to bother you in the middle of the day like this."

"Oh, no problem. I'm just eating my friend. I mean, eating *with* my friend. I don't actually eat people. Salads, I-I eat . . . salad."

My mortified voice faded like the slow drone of a robot losing power. I could feel mortification heat my cheeks in a red-hot blush. People? I don't eat people? My internal voice kept screaming. *Bradley is on the phone! On. The. Phone. I'm going to die! This isn't happening!*

Bradly chuckled and my heart almost dropped out of my ribcage. "I also hope you're not freaked out by me calling so unexpectedly. You gave me your phone number a while ago, but I never used it because we always just use Facebook. I tried messaging you there but you weren't on, so I thought I'd just give this a try."

"No problem," I said weakly.

"I'm just at the bookstore and wanted to grab the book that we agreed to read, but I couldn't—and this is really embarrassing because I'm kind of air-headed about stuff like this—remember what book we decided on."

He laughed, this time sounding sheepish. I glanced up just in time to see Rachelle head across the cafeteria, hands on her ample hips, eyes locked on her prey.

"*Frankenstein.* I-it's *Frankenstein.*"

"Right!" He snapped his fingers in the background. "You'd think I could remember that, right?"

"Oh, no problem."

Call me anytime, lover boy.

"How is your day going?" he asked, and my eyes widened to the size of saucers. Was he actually asking about my day? A boy? And not just *any* boy, but beautiful, broad-shouldered Bradley?

"Busy," I replied once I pulled myself from my stupor enough to realize that an awkward silence had stretched. "Just finished class and I'm eating with my friend Rainbow Brite."

"Your friend is Rainbow Brite?"

"Rachelle!" I cried, realizing my mistake in horror. "I meant Rachelle. She just dresses like Rainbow Brite. She's not actually Rainbow Brite because that's a cartoon, right? She just wears the tube socks and hair ribbon and costume."

He laughed a deep belly laugh this time. "So your friend dresses like Rainbow Brite and wears tube socks?"

"Yes."

I buried my face in my hands and wished I could die.

"Well I can't wait to meet her this summer. Listen, it was great to talk to you, and fun to hear your voice. You sound just like I thought. Anyway, I found the book and need to buy it before I run off to my next class. I'll talk to you later? Maybe tonight?"

I wasn't sure whether I'd imagined the eager sound of his tone, so I tried to pretend like I hadn't heard, but kidded myself. I'd play that phrase over and over again in my mind for the next couple of months.

I'll talk to you later?

"Of course." I swallowed a nervous lump in my throat. "Tonight after work sounds great."

"Excellent. Later, Lex."

The call ended with the sound of a dial tone and my hammering heart. I blinked, stared at the screen, and tried to tell myself it hadn't been a dream. Bradley had actually called me. Called *me,* Lexie Greene, the girl known for her ability to eat ten Taco Bell tacos when she was sad.

"Oh," I whispered, pressing a shaky hand to my face. "Oh, goodness. He called me Lex. He gave me a nickname."

"Nailed it!" Rachelle declared, dropping onto the bench across from me with a thump that rattled both tables. A piece of scrap paper between her fingers floated to the table. "He's taking me to a buffet tonight. Hell yeah."

I smiled weakly, thinking about the irony of her pigging out while I dreamed of going to the gym and working out so hard that I sweated into a puddle on the floor.

Can I talk to you later? Bradley's voice repeated through my mind again. *Maybe tonight?*

Rachelle studied me with a long sigh. "Your mom is right, you know. You really do have a pretty face, Lexie. You should try to date more. Who cares how much we weigh? Big girls are hot, hot, hot. Proof is on the table."

I hardly heard a word she said, glossing over her repetition of the phrase *you have such a pretty face* that Mom always told me growing up, although she always tacked on *but pretty girls aren't overweight.*

"Congrats, Rachelle," I said, thinking of Bradley and his easy laugh. "Sounds like a great time. Let me know how it goes."

Because I have a date of my own.

Chapter 18—Head and Heart

The next week passed in a string of similar days.

School, work, Rachelle spouting off about her recent conquests with the gamer, chat with Bradley at night on Facebook, avoid McKenzie and her constant stream of wedding plans, and fall asleep watching weight loss television.

"It's getting old, don't you think?" I asked Mira Wednesday evening while waiting for Bitsy to finish filling up glasses of ice water in her kitchen. Mira lifted an eyebrow in a silent question. "Counting calories, I mean."

My smart phone glowed in my hand while I punched in my numbers for the day. I hadn't eaten dinner yet—on purpose, of course—and still had three hundred calories left. Another salad for me.

"It got old the first day," Mira replied.

"It was revelatory at first. Who knew pickles didn't have calories? Maybe even there was a sense of adventure in the change, but now it's just annoying. I mean seriously. We have to count everything?"

Mira held up her hands in praise. "Hallelujah, my friend."

Despite my grumblings, counting calories seemed a lot less painful than seeing the scale creep back up again, so I chose the lesser of two evils and forced myself to be honest. Okay, I'd snuck in an extra pat of butter at lunch. So maybe I only had two hundred and fifty calories left.

"Welcome to the third week of the *Health and Happiness Society*," Bitsy declared, handing out water. Her eyes had a subtle hint of redness to them, though it could have just been the poor light in the room. The distant sound of girls shrieking came down the back hall.

"As always, let's get started with the weigh-in and get the worst part over with. I'm going to talk with you today about eating our exercise calories back. Should we or shouldn't we? Mira, you're first. Lexie, you'll be last."

Mira hopped up first wearing a bright blue muumuu with palm trees on it that I hadn't seen since we celebrated Christmas together when I was thirteen. Her face didn't seem as bloated that evening: a definite sign of progress.

By the time my turn came, Mira and one of the men were chatting quietly about the benefits of using an ab roller. "I'd fall right on my face," Mira said when Bitsy called me back.

"Lexie, you're up."

Bitsy walked just behind me down the hall, like a prison guard escorting a criminal. I felt like I'd done something wrong by the time I turned into the small bathroom, and wondered if she knew about my shameful bad day.

"Mira said the two of you had a tough beginning last week," Bitsy said, pressing her lips together in an inscrutable expression I couldn't read. "Want to tell me about it?"

Not on your life.

"Bad day, that's all," I said, sliding out of my flip-flops. I'd worn my lightest black pants and a simple t-shirt. Normally I chose my outfits based solely on how many of my love handles would show, but I didn't care about that as much at the group meetings. All I wanted was lower numbers, baby. Fashion be banned.

"Step on. Let's see if your bad day damaged your scale day."

I closed my eyes and stepped on the scale, feeling like a coward because I didn't want to see the results. Interminable seconds ticked by.

"Well?" Bitsy asked. "Aren't you going to look?"

I peeled one eye open and glanced down. *252.*

Bitsy consulted the clipboard of power that she kept on the sink. "You lost two pounds this week. That's really good for week two, Lexie. Looks like your bad day didn't hurt you too much, though we'll never know, will we?"

A breath of relief escaped me. My eyes moistened just enough to blur my vision. Had I been *that* stressed over this weigh-in? I swallowed, embarrassed at my emotion, and blinked the tears away.

"I binged," I confessed, my head bowed like a child caught with her hand in the figurative cookie jar. "I had a bad day and ate doughnuts and mozzarella sticks and pizza rolls."

Bitsy listened with the same intensity that she did everything, narrowed eyes, face scrunched, deep in thoughts I couldn't even fathom. I wanted her to understand I had only given up once; that I'd picked myself back up and forced myself to keep going. Her militant approval was far more important than I'd realized.

"We all binge at some point," she said with a sigh, and I saw a flicker of something in her eyes. "The important thing is that you learn from it by identifying the steps that led to it."

My forehead ruffled. "What do you mean?"

"Think back on that day. What happened? Why did you eat?"

"Because I always eat," I replied immediately. Her question didn't make any sense. Why wouldn't I eat when I was upset? What else was there to do? I thought about how Mira and I went to the gym that evening, and wondered if that had something to do with it.

"Okay," she drawled, folding her arms over the clipboard. "But what point did you reach that finally made you feel like *enough. I can't handle this without food or sugar.*"

She stared at me so intently that for a moment I lost my train of thought, but slowly picked it back up again. "I was driving home after a bad day, I hadn't eaten because I was late for class, didn't have any money, everything went wrong, and I passed a doughnut shop. I ate so fast that I didn't even enjoy them," I admitted with a grimace. "Then I returned home and Mom was upset with me so I just grabbed a plate of food and hid in the basement."

Bitsy held up one hand with her fingers splayed. "First, you were hungry and hadn't eaten. Second, you were upset about your bad day, didn't know how to deal with it, so you ate something to make you feel better or forget all the bad things. Did it make you forget?"

"No."

"Third," she continued, ticking the fingers off with her other hand. "You were avoiding confrontation with your mother by hiding behind food."

I stared at her in a daze. Never in all my life had I analyzed the motivations behind what I ate. Never had I truly *realized* that there were reasons behind why I ate so much bad—yet scrumptious—food. Hunger or sadness or depression or frustration all seemed easier to deal with when I had a little sugar in me. Sure, I felt good on the sugar high, but never thought to look into why I felt bad in the first place.

"I never thought of it that way," I whispered. Bitsy smirked.

"I know. That's why you're here."

"I did work out afterwards. I felt better."

"Good," she said, startled. "You transferred your focus from food to something healthy. Did it make you feel better?"

"Yes."

"And food didn't?"

"No," I whispered, eyes wide. "It didn't. I guess it . . . it never really does."

"No, it doesn't. Not when it's done for emotional reasons, anyway." Bitsy studied me for a moment. "Do you want to avoid another binge?"

I nodded desperately.

"When you get home, I want you to write down everything that happened from the moment you woke up to the moment you went to sleep that day in a column. Next to it, I want you to write what emotions you were feeling at the time. All of them. Any of them. If it came to your mind, write it down. Look back on other bad binge days you've had and can remember, and write those out. See if you notice a pattern."

The idea of revisiting dark days in my past didn't excite me, but I couldn't deny a touch of curiosity in the assignment. I thought weight loss involved lettuce, calorie restrictions, and drinking lemon water by the gallon. I never imagined the battle had so much to do with my head and heart.

"Okay. I'll do it."

"In the meantime, good job. You still lost two pounds. You've lost seven pounds in the last two weeks, which is really good." She smiled, which softened the intensity around her eyes. "Now comes the hard part: not giving up."

Chapter 19—Loaves and Fishes

The moment Mira dropped me off at home after the weigh-in, I hurried downstairs, waving to McKenzie on my way, and opened my computer. My mind spun so quickly that I ignored the notifications on my Facebook account that could only mean Bradley wanted to talk to me.

Bitsy's advice had seized my mind. While the idea of hashing through emotions to admit an ungainly truth I didn't want to face didn't excite me, I was curious. In fact, I didn't feel relief until I listed every event of that terrible day. In a column next to it, I wrote everything else.

Frustrated with traffic
Ashamed of myself
Depression because I could only think of food
Self-loathing for eating two doughnuts without enjoying them
Self-loathing for needing two doughnuts
Annoyance that I can't stick to a diet
Annoyance that I'm overweight at all
Annoyed that I was hungry
Annoyed that this process is so hard
Angry I'm not good enough for Mom
Angry I'm not my sister

By the time I finished the self-examination, I stared at the blinking cursor on my computer screen and swallowed heavily.

"Good grief," I muttered. Despite having lost two more pounds, I felt a gaping hole inside my chest when I realized the extent of my problems. I wasn't just dependent on food to feel good or deal with a bad day.

I was totally *addicted* to it.

Food had carried me through a turbulent childhood with constant, subtle reminders from my mom that I wasn't skinny enough. Food had bonded me to my dad. Food had seen me through his

75

death. Food had been there when it seemed no one else had. Food also made me depressed and insecure.

Like a songbird from my closet, the secret stash of Ho Ho's and Little Debbie snacks called to me from the black depths.

We always make you happy, they seemed to say. *Remember all the nights we've spent together? How good the chocolate frosting tasted when nothing else felt good in your life?*

And for a moment, I listened.

"*Did* you make me happy?" I asked out loud, tears filling my eyes. "Because I don't feel very happy right now."

Thoughts of my favorite foods danced through my mind for a minute. Chocolate cake. Warm apple pie with cold ice cream. Cupcakes with frosting and doughnuts with sprinkles. At least I'd feel happy for a moment.

I finally stood, walked to the closet, ripped it open, grabbed my stash of happy snacks, and shoved them all into the garbage. Just to be sure I wouldn't eat them, I dumped window cleaner on top.

Exhausted, I collapsed on my bed and fell asleep.

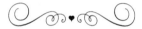

"You all right this morning, Lex?" Mira asked, eyeing me from her place on the elliptical next to mine. The quiet whir of machines and the occasional clank of someone dropping a weight set filled the background. I'd come to be okay with the easy atmosphere of the gym in the morning, although I still couldn't say I looked forward to it.

"Yeah," I said, trying to infuse my voice with sincerity I didn't feel. I didn't want to tell her that I'd dreamed of Fudge Bars chasing me all night long. "Just tired, I think."

Mira kept going on the elliptical, but kept a worried eye on me. I rubbed a hand over my face to wake myself up, still feeling sluggish. Once my intervals finished, I climbed off the machine and trundled over to the water cooler for a drink. Halfway through my cup, a body ran into me, splashing ice water all over my face.

"Oh, sorry! I'm so sorry. I'm such a klutz. I didn't mean to trip into you."

I looked up to find a familiar pair of brown eyes and brown hair, above the usual yoga pants, standing next to me. When I'd first started working out at the gym, she had been with another girl in the weight section. Instead of wearing her straight, silky brunette hair in a braid like normal, she wore it in a loose ponytail today. I saw her at least every other day now, and I wondered if she noticed. Both girls fascinated me. They weren't supermodel skinny, nor were they overweight like me, and they still wore those tight black yoga pants I'd never be brave enough for.

"It's okay," I said, wiping the excess water off my face. "I needed a wake up."

To my surprise, she laughed. Mirth at this early hour seemed overkill in other people, but it fit her. "I really am sorry," she said again. "Getting up this early is awful, don't you think? I can barely walk."

"Yeah, it's getting kind of old." I smiled halfheartedly and stifled the urge to be brutally honest.

I also just figured out that I'm completely addicted to food, can't cope without it, hate waking up knowing I have to count calories, and can't bring myself to love working out, so the gym just really inspires me most mornings.

"I see you here a lot." She reached for a cup and dumped some water inside. "Do you come every morning?"

"Yep. Six days a week now."

"Impressive. I come here four days a week, and that's just about all I can manage."

Her toned body didn't look like it was suffering.

"You look like that and you only work out four days a week?" I blurted out with a sudden surge of courage that made me blush. "Oh, sorry. That wasn't polite, was it?" I mumbled, trying to recover. "I-I guess I just thought that you must work out like twice a day."

"Nah." She waved a nonchalant hand through the air. "I don't have time or energy for that."

"You do all those weights. Surely that takes plenty of energy."

Speaking with strangers wasn't my thing, but this girl didn't seem so bad. She had an easy confidence I envied, like she didn't even care that girls weren't supposed to lift weights. Were they? I didn't understand this new idea. "It must have taken you forever to be able to figure all . . . *that stuff* out."

"Not really. Once I started doing it, I liked it so much I just kept going. It all builds on itself."

"Aren't you going to get jacked?" I asked imitating a body builder pose. "Like super buff for competitions and stuff?"

Her nose wrinkled when she laughed. "No way! I'm not interested in that kind of thing, I just like that it makes me stronger. You could do it too, you know. It's not that bad once you learn how to do it right. We could start you with a kettle bell. Now *that* is a serious workout."

I laughed so hard, and so loud, I drew the attention of two college girls pretending to study on the bikes nearby.

"Me? Do things with weights? Let's just say it's another loaves and fishes miracle from the Bible that I'm here at all."

Her face sobered almost instantly. "Why are you here?"

"To look hot and lose weight like everyone else." My voice lowered with special confidence, thinking that telling her about Bradley would certainly win her over. "I'm meeting this guy in a few months and want to make his jaw drop at my sister's wedding. Not to mention I look like a bloated pink Smurf in my bridesmaid dress."

To my surprise, she didn't look impressed. In fact, she seemed a bit confused, maybe even let down the way Bitsy always looked when she suspected my true motives.

"Oh, I see. Well, if you ever are interested in trying out something new, let me know. I'm here four mornings a week and would love to teach you how to do it." She smiled and stuck out her hand. "I'm Megan."

I hesitated, blinking in disbelief. I wanted to ask her why she was there early in the morning four times a week if not to impress a guy. Why else look hot? Why else slave away counting calories and working out if not to look sexy? I really didn't understand this girl.

"Lexie," I said, taking her hand. "Lexie Greene."

She shook it with a firm grip. "Good to meet you. I hope we can work out together in the future."

She slipped away with a lot more grace than she'd introduced herself, leaving me standing at the water station with an empty paper cup in my hand and what must have been a stunned look on my face. Not knowing what else to do, I returned to the cardio area and got on a treadmill, my mind spinning.

Chapter 20—Kit Kat Calorie Reality

I stared at the shopping cart with an intense feeling of trepidation.

Shopping meant food. Food meant looking at calories. Looking at calories meant learning the truth about foods I loved. No, I really didn't want to know how many calories were in a Fudge Round, thank you very much. Then I couldn't eat them all in innocence next time.

In my world, ignorance was definitely bliss.

"Whoa, Mira. You didn't say anything about going grocery shopping," I said, palms up. "I thought we were just going to get something to eat for breakfast. This is Friday, remember? My day off. Let's not ruin it by subjecting me to the torture of looking at pastries I can't have."

Mira set her Mary-Poppins-sized purse in the front of the cart.

"We need to learn about shopping for healthy food," she said primly, clad in her less-than-subtle bright neon blue workout pants and leg warmers. At least her makeup wasn't equally bright. This time.

"And who is going to teach us how to shop for healthy food?" I asked, eyeing a display of red velvet cookies. Mira had about as much credibility teaching healthy eating as I did teaching about long-distance running.

"I am."

My stomach clenched. I whirled around to find Bitsy stride up next to us and set her mom purse next to Mira's. Like always, she wore a pair of clothes that meant she could have just finished working out. She didn't even break stride.

"Follow me."

I glanced at Mira with a condemning glare, but she smiled irreproachably and toddled forward after our personal drill sergeant. With a sigh, I caved and trudged on, already dreading the next hour.

"When you're shopping," Bitsy began, motioning around her with a sweep of her arms as she moved to the right, "you want to stick as close to the edges of the store as possible. All the processed junk is in the middle. See? The produce is just over here."

We passed a young mother with a new baby as we trailed behind Bitsy like ducks waddling in a row. Normally I didn't come to this part of the grocery store—I consumed plenty of fresh vegetables through the cabbage in my egg rolls, thanks—so walking to the right seemed a bit strange. I always went straight forward, right to the Tostito's.

"Preparation is the key pillar in any dieting strategy," Bitsy began.

Although I heard everything, my eyes snagged on a display of angel food cake and fresh strawberries. *Mmm . . . strawberries with cool whip on top of a pillowy slice of angel food cake. The red sauce would drip off the sides and—*

"—Stick as close to the natural state of the food as you can get, and never shop hungry."

I jerked out of my salivating daydream to find Bitsy glaring at me, hands on her circular hips, eyes narrowed.

"Am I interrupting anything?" she asked me with the arch look of an elementary school teacher.

"No ma'am. Sorry."

"As I was saying . . . you need to have a plan. A list. Train yourself to only get what is on the list. That requires planning and forethought, but just consider those the price of good health and success." She whipped around, headed for a lineup of vegetables. "Now let's talk about organic versus regular produce . . ."

I had just turned to follow when I caught sight of myself in a mirror above the display of lettuce and radishes. Bitsy's voice trailed away. I stared, shocked at what I saw.

My shirt hung like a loose rag off my shoulders.

Like a moth drawn to flame, I ventured forward a few steps, staring at myself. Surely I wasn't imagining the way the shirt hung lower on my arms than it used to, at least to my elbows. My face didn't appear as swollen as it used to either. In fact, I dared to think that my second chin had shrunk. Robotically, I reached my hands down to my thighs and pulled at the fabric.

Loose.

Looser than it had ever been.

A little tremor of excitement ran through me. Sure, I'd lost seven pounds according to the scale, but my clothes showed the progress also. Ecstatic, I whirled around to see Bitsy and Mira studying something green and fluffy. Oh, I'd seen it before in a special frozen chicken cordon bleu. Broccoli.

I shuddered in delight again. *My clothes were loose!* This had never happened before. Not even when I bought new clothes.

"Roast it with a little olive oil," Bitsy was saying as I floated up, humming. "Or steam it with a little lemon pepper seasoning. It's delicious, low calorie, high in fiber, and good for you. Oh, hello Lexie. Are you joining us now?"

Not even Bitsy's disciplinarian tone could bring me down.

"Yes," I sang, spreading my arms wide. "Teach me everything. Take my flab!"

Make me hot, hot, hot for Bradley!

Bitsy sucked in a breath as if about to scold me, but let it out. She straightened as if she'd just come up with a genius diabolical plan.

"Fine," she said. "Take your flab? Let's start by taking a look at the foods you *used* to eat, shall we? I think I can open your eyes a little bit to where all that flab came from."

I followed behind, humming, drifting through the happy clouds of my now skinner self, looking at everything I passed with new eyes.

You won't help me lose weight, I said to a box of chocolate zingers, although my stomach growled at the thought of the rich frosting. *You won't help me fit in a black dress for Bradley,* I thought when I passed a case of Capri Sun. Fruit punch—my favorite. A tower of various Little Debbie snacks stood at the end of one aisle, and I had to avert my eyes and hurry past.

"Little Debbie is not my friend."

"This is a box of breakfast cereal," Bitsy announced, pulling my very favorite from the shelf as if she'd known it was one of my mortal weaknesses. My eyes widened in delight.

"I love that cereal!!" I cried, and Bitsy gave me a suspicious stare. I backed up. "But I haven't had any since I started in the *Health and Happiness Society*, I swear!"

"It's my favorite too," Mira agreed with a sheepish smile. "My husband used to eat it with chocolate milk."

Bitsy's upper lip curled. "Yikes. Chocolate milk? Have you ever looked at the nutrition facts?"

My smile dropped. "No. Why would I do that? Why would you do that? It'll just ruin it forever."

"Let's hope," Bitsy said, and shoved the nutrition label in my face. "Read it for me."

"But—"

"Do you want to be healthy?"

I want to be skinny, I almost said, but seeing the look on her face, held back. Neither Bitsy nor Mira would appreciate my striving for hotness over health. I took the box.

"Ha!" I cried. "There's only one gram of fat per serving! Take that."

"Start at the top. How much cereal in one serving?"

"One cup."

"How many cups do you eat?"

"Honestly?" I queried, eyes narrowed. She rolled her eyes. "Yes."

"Probably two cups per bowl."

"How many bowls?"

I hesitated. "Two . . . or three on a really bad day."

Bitsy didn't even appear phased. "Okay, so you have up to six servings of cereal in one sitting. How many grams of sugar per cup? Grams of sugar, not carbohydrates."

"Twenty-two," I replied hesitantly, which seemed high, but I wasn't *exactly* sure. I'd only been looking at labels for the past two weeks, and mostly just at calories in my desperation to stick to my allotment. What did sugar have to do with calories anyway?

She handed Mira a Kit Kat bar that I hadn't even seen her pick up. "How many grams of sugar in a Kit Kat bar?"

"Twenty-two," she whispered weakly. My eyes popped open.

"What?" I screeched.

"So if I eat two bowls of cereal then I'm really just eating four Kit Kat bars?" Mira asked, mimicking my own incredulousness. Impossible! Kit Kat bars were candy. Cereal had . . . whole grains and stuff.

Bitsy smirked. "In terms of actual sugar grams, yes. Eye opening, isn't it?"

"More like sickening," I muttered, pressing a hand to my stomach. I had no idea that my *healthy cereals* compared to candy bars. Why did it have to taste so good?

"Come on," Bitsy said with a maniacal grin. "Wait until I show you the ingredients in frozen pizza."

Chapter 21—The Machine

When I went to the gym the next morning, my new brunette friend Megan wasn't there. Although I always made a point to smile or wave to her whenever I saw her, now that we'd actually connected, I felt a bit relieved she hadn't shown up. Today I, Lexie Greene, was going to do something I'd never done in my life.

Use a weight lifting machine.

"What are you staring at?" Mira asked, puffing away next to me on the elliptical. Her legs flashed in and out of each other in surprising sequence. Instead of gawking at the newscaster, she'd started paying attention to her workout lately. "You look like you're staking out a chili dog stand or a place to drop a nuke."

Not a nuke, just my body.

"I don't know." I shrugged nonchalantly, my feet whirring in the elliptical next to hers. We'd been going to the gym for weeks—which felt more like an eternity—and I had started to dread the same routine of bike, elliptical, treadmill. "Just thought I'd try out something different today. You know that weight loss TV show I watch? The episode last night said that you should change up your routine if you start getting bored."

"Try swimming."

I snorted. "Swimsuit in public? Not on your life."

She cocked an eyebrow. "What else is there for people like you and me?"

"Like a weight lifting machine."

"You're going to try one of those?" she asked, swinging her head to the other side of the gym where a young man was pushing some sort of bar into the air with painful grunts.

"Yeah, well, I'm just getting bored, you know? I either wog on the treadmill or ride this thing. Don't you just want to change it up sometimes?"

She mumbled something suspiciously close to *all I want is a Pepsi*, so I left her to her mutterings and scouted out the options again. Surely it couldn't be *that* bad, could it?

"What if you hurt yourself?" she asked. "You have no idea what you're doing on those things. Then you wouldn't be able to work out, and then you wouldn't lose weight."

And then you'll meet Bradley looking like this, my brain finished. I rolled my eyes and shoved those thoughts away. "I'm not going to hurt myself."

"Yes you are."

"Look, it's not like I'm going to do those free weights that Megan does," I cried, shuddering at the thought. "They look too complicated and I'd probably drop one on my face. These machines don't look so bad."

"Weights will make you all jacked up and buff like a man."

"Megan said they don't and I trust her. I'm going to do it, Mira. I'm determined. I'm also bored out of my mind watching a rerun of *Jeopardy.* They never have anything good on. What happened to *Golden Girls?*"

She pressed her lips to one side of her face in a dubious gesture that solidified my determination.

"Oookay," she sang. "Can't wait to see this."

Resolute, I stopped the elliptical and clambered off. The tip of my sneaker caught the foot pad and I stumbled, but caught myself by hanging off the handlebar until I could regain my feet. Mira snorted. I avoided her judgmental gaze by straightening my clothes and walking, head high, to the other side of the gym. I stopped at the indoor track that the sweaty Asian man looped around every morning.

I'd never crossed the track before.

It felt like a moment out of a warped version of *West Side Story.* When I finally walked across, I found myself swimming in a veritable jungle of iron, rack, and weight. I crossed my arms in front of me, suddenly nervous. Mira was right. I had no idea how to use any of these. When I glanced over my shoulder, she was intently watching, a half-smirk on her face.

"Well," I said, finding my courage again. "I can't let Mira think she's right."

I strode up to the first machine I saw and studied it. A few badly drawn pictures explained how to use it. Looked like a shoulder exercise. All I had to do was sit down and push it upwards.

Too easy.

I sat down, gripped the handles, and pushed up, but it didn't budge. I tried again. Nothing.

"Broken!" I cursed under my breath. It would be my luck to find the broken machine amongst this sea of others. The sound of someone clearing their throat came next to me.

"You might just need to change the weight," a voice said. "Looks like it's set at a hundred pounds right now. Unless you feel like you can do a shoulder press at a hundred, that's not going to move."

I glanced through the tangle of cord and machine to see a pair of blue eyes belonging to an employee cleaning the machine next to me with a spray bottle and a rag. He smiled in the tight, restrained way that meant he was trying not to laugh.

"Oh," I said. "I hadn't actually thought of that."

"It's right there." He motioned with a nod to a tower of square plates with numbers on them.

"Right, yeah. I was just . . . just about to do . . . that."

"And you're sitting in it wrong. Your back is supposed to be against the backboard. You face out. Not in."

I stared at the backrest and wondered if he'd clean up the mess I made by melting with embarrassment. *What am I doing here?* I thought. *I have no idea how this world functions. I don't belong.*

My face flared so hot I could have cooked a hot dog on it. *Hot dog,* I thought, feeling a sudden urge to eat one. *With lots of relish and mustard. It tastes so good. I definitely belong with a hot dog. That's more my thing.*

Drill sergeant Bitsy's voice broke through my mind from our last weigh-in. *You didn't know how to deal with it, so you ate.*

My last binge had started from me being in a situation where I felt strong emotions that I wanted to forget, just like this one. I opened my mouth to ask for his help but hesitated. Would he laugh at me? Would these machines support my weight? Did I look stupid trying to get skinny when I clearly wasn't?

The sudden deluge of fears flipped a switch in my mind, and suddenly I was dreaming of a stack of pancakes and bacon. Dripping butter, warm syrup, and a tart glass of orange juice on the side.

No! I won't do this.

"Excuse me," I asked, though it came out feeble and quiet. "Would you mind explaining how to use this? Or any of these? I don't know how many . . . uh . . . times to do it."

He brightened. "How many reps to do, you mean?"

"Sure, yeah. *Reps.*"

His eyes narrowed in thought. I fought to keep myself from crossing my arms over my body in self-conscious fear.

"Have you ever used a weight lifting machine before?" he asked.

Do I look like I have? I wanted to snap, but shook my head instead. "No. This is a first for me." I glanced at the tower of weight plates. "Obviously."

He laughed at that. "Of course," he said. "I'd love to show you. In fact, we have workout sheets over here. You can just keep them in the file and write down what you do each time you come so you can keep track. Let me grab a clipboard and I'll explain it."

And so, for the next twenty minutes of the morning, the nice man named Jeff and I moved through the weight lifting machines with methodical ease. He explained while I demonstrated, and by the end, the whole jungle didn't seem so intimidating. A bit scary perhaps. The muscles in my legs and arms felt strange, like someone kept pulling on the different ends, but it wasn't an entirely *unpleasant* experience.

"I wrote you up a few workout samples to try out," Jeff said once we'd finished the end of the tour. He extended the clipboard to me. "See if you like them. Try it in reps of eight first and go from there. Mixing weight with cardio is a really good way to look toned."

I took the clipboard. "You're certain that lifting weights won't make me look like a man?"

"No. Not at this low intensity. Women who look like men know they're going to, and they work hard for it. This will just tone you up."

I hesitated. The words he'd written all looked like a jumbled mess to me. I almost snorted when I saw the word *abs* listed among them.

Right. Like I had abs.

"Thank you, Jeff," I said, sticking out my hand. "I really appreciate you showing me around."

"No problem. I'm here every morning, so I'm sure we'll run into each other."

He moved off to help another client, leaving me standing in the field of machines like a lost human in a robot world. I only had a few more minutes left at the gym, which meant I'd only really worked out for fifteen minutes. But I *felt* as if I'd conquered something great.

"Looks like you'll have to come back tonight," Mira said over my shoulder, dabbing sweat off her face with a towel. "Since you spent the morning flirting with that guy."

I stared at her in shock. "I wasn't flirting. I was taking charge of my own life by learning how to work out."

Mira's eyebrows lifted in surprise. "Yes," she drawled with a slow smile. "I guess you were, weren't you?"

I slowly grinned back. "Yeah. Yeah, I was."

And it felt great.

Chapter 22—It's On

Bradley: **Hey Lex!** *I haven't seen you online for a day or two. Felt kind of weird not IMing with you. Are you enjoying your Sunday?*

Lexie: *Sorry! I had to work late last night (an Irish pub on Saturday night is insane) and slept in today because Sunday is my only day off from the gym.*

Bradley: *You work out?*

Lexie: *Uh . . . yeah! I'm not super good at it, but I go. Does that count?*

Bradley: *Awesome! How have we not talked about this before? What's your favorite thing to do when you work out? I love lifting. I kind of suck at running, but I do it because of practice. We should work out together after your sister's wedding!*

My eyes widened. Work out with Bradley? In all my boob-stomach-bouncing-glory? I scrambled for something to say. "Divert," I whispered, frantically typing. "Divert, divert, divert!"

Lexie: *Unless you're totally hammered. They're having an open bar.*

Bradley: *Nah. I'm not big on the alcohol scene to be honest.*

Lexie: *Of course not. Well, er, how do I say this? My run is more like . . . a wog.*

Bradley: *I just snorted Diet Dr Pepper through my nose. A wog? What is that?*

My eyes fell to the half-full plastic bottle of Diet Dr Pepper next to my computer. "We are soul mates, Mr. Bradley."

The latest episode of my weight loss TV show played in the background, a constant reminder for me not to go upstairs and snack on

90

the four slices of buttered wheat toast that I couldn't stop thinking about. It would be so easy, and yet . . .

I sighed and took another swig of pop, eyeing the plate of celery and bottle of water next to it. I'd get to them eventually.

Lexie: *A wog is a walk/jog combo.*

Bradley: *Ha! I love it. Hey, I've been reading Frankenstein.*

I breathed a sigh of relief. Ah, safety.

Lexie: *Oh? What are you thinking so far?*

Bradley: *I have to say, the beginning is pretty intense. Not sure I'd want to go north on a voyage to the North Pole, so lonely.*

I grinned, unable to help myself. He'd barely started the book!

Lexie: *Is that as far as you've gotten? The letters at the beginning?*

Bradley: *. . . maybe . . . *sheepish smile**

Lexie: *Just keep going. It's a great story.*

Bradley: *How is the internship thing going?*

Lexie: *Good. Slow work, but I work on a few things for it a little bit every day. My advisor is helping me out.*

Bradley: *Can I ask you a really random question?*

Lexie: *Sure.*

Bradley: *Do you have any recent pictures of yourself?*

My brain seized in terror. Recent pictures? No! I never took pictures! The proportions my chins to the rest of my body drew far too much attention.

"Oh dear," I murmured. "Oh . . . dear."

How could I get him off this dangerous path? This had turned into walking through a field of land mines. Admitting I went to the gym six times a week frightened me enough; what if he found out that I worked out so much because I had so much weight to lose? He'd stop talking to me completely.

Lexie: I don't really have a new picture, no.

Bradley: Mostly curious.

Lexie . . . yeah . . . not a big fan of looking at my own face, you know?

Bradley: But you have a beautiful face.

My stomach flipped in a painful way. "You haven't seen the rest of me, Bradley boy," I muttered, grabbing a spear of celery and crunching through it with a vengeance. I pretended it tasted like a Pringle and it didn't seem so bad.

Lexie: Ah, thanks. That's very sweet. Most of the pictures on Facebook are probably before my dad died, I think.

And before I gained at least forty pounds and found my second chin. I chugged half the bottle of water.

Bradley: yeah, the pictures say they're at least two years old. Is your hair still that long? C'mon, just one pic! A new one just for me. You can send it in the message. You don't even have to post it for everyone else.

Lexie: Well, I haven't taken any pictures recently because I'm on this healthy kick.

I closed my eyes and hung my head in defeat. "Healthy kick? What kind of response is *that*, Lexie? ARGH!"

Bradley: I need to be on a healthy kick. College life is brutal. I don't even have plates. Are you dieting?

Lexie: Er . . . yes. I guess you could call it a diet? I'm not allowed to eat Little Debbie snacks, which means I'm on a diet, right?

My stomach cramped. Even my pathetic attempt at infusing humor in the comment didn't help soften my new reality.

Bradley knew.

The cat was out of the bag. I was on a diet, which meant I needed to lose weight, which meant I wasn't perfect and Bradley was going to totally give me up. The cursor blinked endlessly while I waited for his response. My heart sat in my throat, pending his sure-to-be-painful rejection. He'd sign off in disgust any minute now.

Lexie isn't perfect, is what he must have been thinking. *She's overweight, not attractive, and can't control her craving for food. That's why she's on a diet. Obviously.*

> Bradley: That's great! Maybe we could eat healthy together! My roommate and I are the worst and I'm going to pay for it once the season starts. What do you think?

My eyes nearly popped out of my head. "That's great?" I screeched. "WHAT?"

It took a few moments for my heart rate to settle back down and my mind to comprehend what this strange change in the conversation meant. Bradley didn't reject me for my diet? He didn't automatically realize that something was wrong with me and I wasn't a perfect beach bunny? I stared at the screen, completely unaware of how to proceed.

> Lexie: You want to eat healthy together?
>
> Bradley: Yeah. I could always use some help being more healthy. I'm not a freshman, but I think I found the freshman fifteen again. :D So how do you do it? Do you count calories? Eat only certain stuff? Avoid dessert? Where should I start?
>
> Lexie: Uh . . . I guess I wasn't expecting this. Some people get all weird when you admit you're on a diet. Yeah, I guess I do all of that.
>
> Bradley: Why would people get weird about it? I admire anyone who is working to be healthy because I'm terrible about sweets and carbs. Seriously. It would be embarrassing to tell you how much I can pack away in a single meal.

I rolled my eyes. "Don't play this game with me, Bradley. I'll match you sumo eater for sumo eater, buddy."

Bradley: Knowing that you're passing on dessert will help me do the same. What do you do for workouts?

I stretched my arms above my head, which felt sore from the weight machines I'd used yesterday. Mira and I had stayed at the gym twenty minutes longer than usual because I had enjoyed the variation that weight machines gave to my workout so much.

Lexie: A lot of cardio, and just started using some of the weight machines.

Typing it out—as if I *really* knew what I was talking about when it came to exercise—made me feel like one of the cool kids for a second. "Yeah," I said arrogantly. "I work out."

Bradley: This is great. I'm excited. Now I have motivation to be healthy thanks to you. Okay, well, I gotta go. I have a pop quiz tomorrow I need to study for. Keep it up at the gym. We have a running date in five months.

I glanced at the calendar on my wall with a little smile. He hadn't rejected me— yet—so maybe I could get in enough shape to wog with him. I grabbed my water bottle and chugged the rest.

Lexie: It's on.

"You didn't lose any weight this week."

I stared at Bitsy without comprehension, blinking at least four times before the words sank in.

"I'm sorry. Can you repeat that?"

"You didn't lose any weight this week, Lex. Sorry, but sometimes that happens. Just keep going and it'll come off."

Bitsy ushered me off the scale with a flapping motion, and I stepped onto my flip-flops, stunned. She marked a big fat zero on her clipboard of power.

"I don't understand," I replied, quickly pulling my hoodie back over my body. "How can I just . . . how can I not lose weight? I've been working so hard. I counted every single calorie. I started lifting weights!"

"You've had a couple of good weight loss weeks, so your body didn't lose this week. It doesn't have to be a big deal. So it was an off week? You'll have them."

Her laissez-faire reaction to this horrific tragedy intensified my anxiety. Why didn't drill sergeant Bitsy care that I hadn't met my goal? Why wasn't she yelling at me and telling me to do push-ups?

"I need to lose every week," I said with a mild feeling of panic. Ever since my last conversation with Bradley, I'd been on a roll. Working out every day. Counting each calorie. Drinking water until I nearly peed myself. To not lose weight? Injustice! "I'm on a deadline. I can't afford *off weeks.*"

Bitsy eyed me with intense suspicion. "What kind of deadline?"

My steam faltered for a moment. "A self-imposed deadline."

"Your sister's wedding?"

"Yes!" I replied, weak with relief that I wouldn't have to mention Bradley. "And the ugliest hot pink dress in the world, if you must know. Every pound that doesn't come off my body is going to be swathed in tulle." I slapped my stomach with both hands. "It's gotta go."

Not to mention I just challenged the love of my life to go for a run with me before the wedding, and he accepted without fear of failure like me.

Bitsy pursed her lips, looking so stern and strict that for a moment I felt relieved. Here it was: the lecture. She was going to tell me how to fix myself so that I could be hawt, hawt, hawt for Bradley.

"This is about that guy you like isn't it?" Bitsy asked. My eyes widened. She must have taken it as confirmation because she continued without encouragement. "Mira told me about your obsession with him although you haven't met yet. Is that why you're part of the *Health and Happiness Society?* Are you worried about losing weight for him?"

"Well . . . I mean, I'm sure it's for myself too but he plays a big . . . uh . . . a big part in my motivation."

Her carefully and painfully plucked eyebrows furrowed over her eyes. She wore her usual workout outfit, one that made it seem like this lifestyle was so easy for people like her. Like the rest of us, Bitsy had been losing weight as well, probably more than anyone although she never said numbers. It showed. Her face appeared thinner, her clothes a little baggy, and a bit of definition had come into her arms. She still didn't smile much, and despite working so hard toward a goal with relative success, didn't seem much happier by it.

"Losing weight is about *you,* not some guy. If you're only doing this for Bradley then you're doing it for the wrong reason. Trust me. Working hard to please someone else, instead of yourself, never brings happiness."

When a haunted glimmer appeared in her eyes, I wondered about her life and marriage. I'd never met her husband. Except for pictures of her two daughters, I didn't see photos of him anywhere.

"Anyway," she drawled, turning away to pull open the bathroom door and let me escape from the disappointment of the pastel prison. "Just keep that in mind."

I opened my mouth to reply, but she had already started down the hall, guards firmly in place and mouth set. I shook my fist at the scale.

"You and I will meet again in one week," I growled, snapping the light off. "One week."

"Can I confess something to you?" I asked Rachelle the next evening while wiping down the bar at Lucky's. Except for two patrons sitting at the end with Pat, cursing a sportscaster that *clearly had never watched sports in his life,* the pub was nearly empty. I reached under the cabinet to refill the straw container.

"Sure."

She dipped a french fry into a shiny blob of ketchup, and my stomach growled. What I wouldn't give for the warm, mealy texture of a salted french fry! I shoved the thoughts away when I saw the scale in my mind from last night again. *252.* Seeing the same number as the week before had nearly crushed me.

It wouldn't happen again.

I straightened up and focused my attention on refilling the straws so I wouldn't have to look in Rachelle's eyes. She looked normal tonight; if normal could apply to a girl like Rachelle. Instead of a costume, she wore her hair in two pigtails and dressed in a pair of ratty jeans with holes in the knees. Without lavish makeup on her face, I almost didn't recognize her.

"I joined a dieting group."

The words exploded from my mouth like they'd been kept there under pressure. The French fry paused midway to her mouth, then resumed. She chewed and shrugged.

"Yeah, I figured as much."

I recoiled. "What?"

"You never eat anymore." She gestured to the empty spot in front of me. "We used to both eat our own plate of fries—sometimes two—whenever I came to visit you. Now you're just drinking Diet Dr Pepper like it's going to save your life."

"The caffeine takes away some of my appetite," I said self-consciously. "How long have you known?"

"Since the day of the salad in the cafeteria. Fateful moment."

"That long?"

"I'm that good."

"And you don't care?"

She rolled her eyes. "Why would I care? You worry way too much about what other people think of you, Lexie Greene. Do your thing, whatever it is. If you want to be fat, be fat. If you want to lose weight, lose weight. It's not a big deal either way. You shouldn't make your decisions based on what other people think of your life."

Rachelle finished her statement with another chomp. I slurped a piece of ice out of my glass and chewed on that instead of snatching a matchstick of deep-fried goodness for myself. Telling Rachelle the truth felt good. Her casual indifference seemed almost like too much to ask for.

"Just don't expect me to diet with you," she said, shaking a fry in my face. "Because that gamer guy didn't work out, so the only love affair left in my life is food, and it does a fantastic job of comforting on a cold winter day."

"The gamer is gone?"

The relationship hadn't much hope from the beginning.

"Nah. He was kind of weird. He put mustard on everything."

"Don't worry. I won't pull you to the dark side."

Relieved to have my secret in the open between us, I tossed the rag in the sink and leaned on my hands. "Now I want to tell you about what Bradley said the other night."

She perked up. "Boy gossip? Spill."

I told her everything about our conversation, his strange response to finding out about my diet, and finally the challenge to exercise with him when he came for the wedding.

"I don't know, Lex. Bradley seems too good to be true. I mean, really? What kind of college guy doesn't care if you're dieting?"

"I don't know," I admitted reluctantly. She'd just voiced the very fear I had myself.

"Be careful. He might be a total jerk that's going to break your heart."

"Or he might be a lot of fun." I hated the hope that lingered in my own voice. "Maybe he's just a good guy."

She rolled her eyes.

"Maybe. I'm not sure I believe in the *good guy* anymore, especially not where imperfect chubby girls are concerned." She slid off the stool and slung her backpack over her shoulder. "All right, I need to go. Thanks for the fries. I'll see you at lunch tomorrow."

Rachelle waddled out the door, casting a flirtatious smile to a middle-aged man, before disappearing into the snowy winter night. I cleaned up her plate, wiped down the area, refilled my pop with ice water, and sank into deeper thoughts.

Chapter 24—Girl Time

By the time that weekend rolled around, I hadn't made a single mistake.

I recorded every single calorie, drank enough water to hydrate a whale, and worked out every morning. My sweatpants had started to get baggy through the legs, which I hardly dared acknowledge for fear I imagined it. Tying the waistband so my pants stayed on—something I had never had to do in my life—meant a beautiful thing was finally starting to happen.

Still, I avoided the mirror when possible. What if I didn't see physical results? My motivation would be crushed. Leaning into *chosen denial* seemed like the easier option.

When I woke up on Saturday morning at six, I started going through the motions of getting ready for the gym like I would on a weekday. Mira and I had plans to go just before lunch, but I figured sooner wouldn't hurt. The sting of seeing *252* kept haunting my dreams. Even the gym would be better than facing a new string of nightmares.

Maybe.

"Hey," I said to myself while slipping my frayed tennis shoes on, "at least I didn't dream about food last night."

An eery quiet met me at the gym. Most people probably chose the wisest route and stayed home in their warm beds. I started my workout with my gaze averted; I felt like I wore a beacon on my back that drew every pair of eyes to me. Without Mira at my side as another big-girl-in-arms, I would seem particularly overweight. The thought made me self-conscious. Was *everyone* staring at me on the bike? Was my stomach sticking out too much? I'd worn my biggest shirt. But . . . wait. . . yep. I was definitely the biggest girl in the room.

Ugh.

I ducked my head into a magazine and tried to convince myself that I could disappear for twenty minutes, not unlike one of those birds that puts their head in the sand. My life had been spent with my metaphorical head in the sands of denial. Twenty more minutes wouldn't kill me.

"Lexie, right?"

I had just stepped away from filling my water bottle at the cooler before heading home—the gym was just too awkward to face by myself without the comfort of Mira at my side—when Megan approached, brown braid swinging, a slight smile on her face.

"Yeah," I said in surprise. "Good memory. How are you?"

She unscrewed the lid on an old Gatorade bottle to fill it up. "As good as can be expected." She gave me a wry smile, but a tinge of fatigue lingered in her slightly red eyes. "I don't normally see you here on Saturday mornings. Why are you up so early?"

"That's a really good question."

To my surprise, she laughed. "I guess that's the question to ask all of us, huh?" she said over the tinkling sound of water filling her bottle. "We must be exceptionally dedicated to a healthy life."

Or desperate. I'm thinking desperate.

"Yeah. Maybe." How quickly could I duck away? The safety of my basement lair beckoned.

"I suppose there are worse reasons to wake up early," Megan said with a friendly smirk, straightening up when her bottle finished filling. Her forehead wrinkled. "Hey, I just finished. Are you done too?"

"Uh, yes. I was just on my way home."

She motioned to a blonde girl in the corner stacking a few black plates on a stand. "That's my friend Dana. We normally go out for breakfast after a workout, but she has to work early so she can't go. Want to come with me?"

I must have panicked like a deer in the headlights because she gave me a reassuring smile. "Don't have to!" she clarified, holding her hands up. "But I thought it might be fun. You seem great."

I swallowed. *Megan* wanted to be friends with me. Confident, self-assured, imperfect-but-didn't-notice-it Megan. "Really?" I heard myself asking. "But you hardly know me."

She waved that off. "I know you like to work out."

"Ha ha . . . no. I hate working out. It's nothing more than a desperate attempt at finding a new reality for my life."

Her eyes crinkled when she laughed again, a full belly laugh that made her tip her head back and put a hand on her stomach. I couldn't imagine how I'd suddenly become funny overnight. Or had I always had a sense of humor, I just hadn't known it?

The idea blew my mind.

"Aren't we all? You don't have to go, but it could be a fun way to start a Saturday. Besides," a wry, nearly bitter tone slipped into her voice, "My boyfriend just broke up with me. I could use some girl time."

My mouth dropped to the floor. "Who would break up with you?"

"Plenty of guys," she replied, her jaw tense. "Trust me. You interested in breakfast?"

Interested? Was she kidding? Of course I wanted to eat with her! Outside of Rachelle, I'd never had anyone ask me for girl time. Or any time for that matter. Not that I really encouraged friendships as a general rule, anyway, so the great unknown mass of potential friends weren't exactly at fault. Eating breakfast sounded perfect except for the annoying little detail that had taken over my life.

"I . . . I'm dieting," I blurted out, and cringed. Megan didn't need to know I was dieting. Likely, she didn't care. If Rachelle hadn't cared, why would Megan? Still, I felt dumb saying it, doubting that Megan had ever had to go on a diet in her life.

"So?"

"Well," I stammered, "I can't eat out while I'm on a diet."

"Sure you can."

I scoffed. "That kind of stuff isn't allowed. In general, I've found that I'm not supposed to eat foods that I enjoy."

She chuckled. "Then we need to get you out more. There's lots of yummy healthy food out there."

"Ha! Sure. I'll believe that when I see it. But thanks for the offer." My shoulders slumped in disappointment. I'd been perfect on my calories and exercise ever since weigh-in, and feared I'd throw off all my mojo if I even *smelled* butter or maple syrup. "It really would have been fun."

Megan's head tilted to the side as if she were confused. "Are you really on that strict of a diet? Because I'm sure we could find something for you."

"Well, I can eat food I guess . . . it's just . . . what can I get that's healthy at IHOP?"

Her nose wrinkled. "IHOP? Gross! We aren't going to go to IHOP. That's not even real food. That's just processed white flour. We'll go to a small place down the road. My friend owns it. I promise, there's plenty of healthy food."

My resolve slowly crumbled. "Bitsy would kill me."

"Who's Bitsy?"

"My drill sergeant." I brushed it off when she raised an eyebrow in question.

"C'mon," she said. "Just try it. If we don't see anything that you can eat on this mysterious diet, we'll go somewhere else until we find food that you can have. We'll grab some fruit at the grocery store if we have too. Sound okay?"

"You'd do that just to eat breakfast with me?"

"Of course. We're practically workout buddies. Let's go."

I followed her to the exit against my better judgment. It wasn't that I didn't trust Megan. Of any human, certainly she'd understand the need for eating healthy. Going out with Rachelle would have guaranteed my failure for the day and an imminent binge. Megan? No. At least . . . I didn't think so. I wasn't all that used to making friends. But I hadn't even stepped foot in a restaurant since the fateful Donut Binge weeks before. Would I have the strength to turn down a dish of sugary sweetness? I didn't have willpower.

I never had.

Drawing in a deep breath, I steeled myself for the inevitable, certain I was just about to break my three-day streak of perfection.

Chapter 25—The Tiki Hut

Megan took me to her friend's restaurant for breakfast after our workout on Saturday morning, all right.

Only she took me to a grass hut.

We walked into a small restaurant that closely resembled the inside of a tiki shack, one I'd expect to see on the side streets of an island somewhere. Torches burned up the path, flickering to island music that sounded like seashells playing in the background. Not that I'd been to any island, of course. Islands had a high swimsuit expectation, and the world wasn't ready for all the cottage cheese my thighs had to offer. The farthest I'd been from my little town had been through the television.

Dad and I had been cheap explorers.

"They serve clean food here," Megan explained, flinging a backpack over her shoulder. I'd driven over because she walked to the gym—a concept I could barely wrap my head around—and held my awkward little handbag on my wrist. How did she attain such casual ease while I managed to make a handbag look frumpy? "They get most of their stuff local, and all their produce is organic. They don't have any of that added crap."

She chose a side table before I could ask what she meant by 'added crap' and 'clean food' as opposed to dirty. A man with dreadlocks and a surfing shirt glanced up from his place behind a register in the back. Once he recognized Megan, he grinned in a way that made me think he'd probably been smoking some of the grass decorating the fringes of the restaurant. Other customers clustered around tables, creating a low, quiet symphony.

"Megan, Megan," he said, loping over with a dopey grin on his face. "It's been a few weeks."

"Hey Cooper. This is my friend Lexie. We just came from the gym."

"Hey, Lex."

While I didn't find Cooper's scruffy hair at all appealing or attractive, I still felt flattered by his casual use of my name. So flattered I forgot to respond and just smiled like I didn't know what was going on. He gestured to the menus already in front of us.

"What are you gals wanting?"

Megan didn't even have to look. "The mango pineapple smoothie with coconut milk and the omelet with goat cheese and bacon." It rolled off her tongue with all the grace of a smooth waterfall. Clearly, this hadn't been the first time she'd eaten here.

"Of course. And you, Lady Lexie?"

I scrambled frantically, my eyes skimming the menu. Chicken sausage? Roasted red pepper omelets? How many calories? Everything sounded so delicious. My stomach wouldn't stop rumbling. I couldn't make a decision so fast! What if I broke my diet again?

And what the heck was *kale?*

"Give her a second, Coop," Megan said. "She's never been here before. But bring her a blackberry kale smoothie for starters on me." She winked at me. "It's my favorite."

He glided away, leaving an earthy fragrance behind.

"Thanks. I haven't eaten out since I . . . well that's not important and—"

"The calories are included on the menu," she said, pointing out a small bold font at the bottom of each dish description that I hadn't noticed in my panic.

"Whoa!" I called in shock. What a novel idea! "That's so cool!"

"And don't worry. Everything you see here is clean."

Images of food rolling around on dirt floors and pigs in mud mires flipped through my mind. Bitsy had used the phrase *clean eating* a few times, but I hadn't really known what it meant. Likely it had something to do with washing fruit before eating it.

"What exactly do you mean by *clean eating?* As opposed to dirty eating, anyway."

She had the presence of mind not to act too startled, though I could see a flicker of it in her eyes.

"Clean eating is avoiding preservatives, additives, and eating food as close to natural as possible. A lot of restaurants add MSG or salt or their food is processed beforehand and they just warm it up. Restaurants like this start from scratch and keep everything natural.

The smoothie that he brings you isn't going to taste like most smoothies you're used to because there isn't ice cream or added sugar. If they do add sugar, they use honey, because it's more natural. The meat they get is local and isn't fed antibiotics or unhealthy diets to fatten them up for butchering."

"Seriously?"

She smiled in the patient, amused way a kindergarten teacher would regard a small child. "Seriously."

"Do people feed animals antibiotics?"

"Among other things."

"Why are preservatives bad? I mean, don't they keep the food edible?"

Megan grimaced. "Ugh. Don't get me started. Some food preservatives used in the US are banned in other countries because the ill effects on health are so bad."

"Really?"

"I believe that being healthy isn't just about exercising," she said with a little shrug. "I think it's about being healthy in *all* ways, and that means taking care of my body with the food I eat. That's why I don't do diets that require me to drink a certain shake or eat a certain meal bar. I eat clean because it makes me feel good."

I stared at her in shock.

Being healthy means taking care of my body with the food I eat.

Not knowing how to respond, I ducked my head back into the menu for a chance to think. Wasn't healthy just being skinny and tan? Eating salads? Wasn't healthy determined by jean size?

By the time Cooper showed up with our smoothies, I'd received a crash course in other preservatives to avoid—which effectively ruined Fanta and bacon for me—and had finally decided on just mimicking Megan's breakfast choice

"Is that why you work out so much?" I asked when Cooper had gone. "Because it's healthy?"

"Of course. Isn't that why you do it?"

"Not really."

Her eyebrows fell into a question, so I rushed to explain.

"You see, there's this guy named Bradley. . ."

She listened without saying a word while I laid the truth bare, telling her everything, from the shame of my constant need to eat, to counting calories so I felt good enough for Bradley. When I finished, she just stared at me, blinking.

"I'm just . . . I'm scared that after all my work I still won't measure up. That I won't be good enough for Bradley."

I ended feeling small and insecure and vulnerable. Megan let out a long breath.

"You don't need Bradley's or anyone's approval of your looks to be happy or love yourself. Did you know that?"

Happy without outside approval? It seemed odd. How else would I know I was pretty unless someone else told me? She'd just introduced a foreign concept, and I didn't know how to grapple with it.

"Uh . . . I didn't . . . I mean—"

I slurped at my drink, startled when the smoothie tasted fresh and light, without a shock of sweetness. The lacking slap of sugar meant the blackberry flavor came out strong. Megan took pity on me with a smile.

"Just think about it. Searching for an outside ideal is never going to make you happy on the inside."

"So what's going on with your boyfriend?" I asked, eager to move away from myself as a topic of conversation. My brain swirled in mad clouds of confusion and excitement.

She sighed. "It's a long story. Suffice it to say that most of my dating ventures end up in disaster. They break it off because I'm just *too intense* or *too motivated*. I think I scare most of them, so after a few months, they back off." She chased down a piece of ice to chew on. "So we broke up."

"What? They're scared?"

She smirked at my confusion. "I know. It doesn't make sense. I just . . . I can't find a guy that likes the same things I do. Most of them are intimidated by me."

"But you're confident and perfect."

"Not perfect. Not even close. But confidence is sometimes a curse, at least in dating. I know what I want. I'm just not convinced it's out there."

I would have given my left thigh to be half of the girl that Megan was—although I was willing to wager my left thigh probably weighed half as much as Megan. To hear her left me wondering whether I even wanted to venture into the dating world. Bradley would certainly never be intimidated by me.

"Did you care for your ex-boyfriend?" I asked.

"Yeah. Yeah, I did. But he still wasn't really what I really wanted. It's like all of them are doomed from the beginning."

Cooper returned with two steaming plates of food. Instead of being overloaded with piles of eggs and syrup and butter, a modest omelet sat in the middle. When I tried my first bite of nitrate-free bacon, I chewed in surprise. Megan grinned, wiping the previous melancholy from her gaze.

"Tastes better, doesn't it?"

"Yeah," I said with a smile. "Yeah, it really does."

♥
Chapter 26—Forget Pie
♠

After Megan and I finished our healthy, preservative-free breakfast, I left the organic tiki hut restaurant puzzling over two things.

1. I'd just left a place of food without overstuffing myself. In fact, I didn't feel sick or bloated or hungry or unsatisfied or euphoric on a food high. I just felt . . . normal.

2. Megan had just introduced an entirely new concept into my life: eating healthy and exercising just because it was the right thing to do.

Say what?

Work out for motivation outside of meeting Bradley? It didn't make a lot of sense at first. After dropping Megan off where she lived in a tiny little cottage next to a big house, I drove on autopilot, my mind whirring. Mom and Kenzie were at home, and although I loved them, I knew they'd pick up on my glum mood like mini satellites and start asking questions. The last thing I wanted to deal with was two weepy women and a fridge full of food that would surely beckon me, so I just kept driving.

Twenty minutes later, I found myself parked in front of the Rose Vine Cemetery. My heart pounded in my chest, making me feel sick. I hadn't been here in far too long.

Far too long.

The early morning grounds remained empty. My old tennis shoes left imprints on the patches of snow left behind from the last winter storm, flat, yellowed grass looked like someone had been laying on it for too long. It smelled like dirt and old snow.

Like Dad, his grave was nothing out of the ordinary. Mom had insisted on a picture of a wreath of flowers on his gravestone, even though we all knew he wouldn't have liked it. But I'd sided with Mom, and said that it was what he would have wanted. Even then, I was beginning to learn that dying was a business for the living, not the dead.

A few straggling vines and a discarded straw wrapper had become entangled near his name. I cleared the debris, tucking the straw wrapper into my pocket so it wouldn't litter this quiet little haven.

"Hey Dad," I said quietly, feeling ashamed. It had been a while since I'd come out to see him. Although he wasn't here, knowing that his body rested in this spot made him feel a bit closer. In that moment, I needed it. Dad had always been my best friend. The eater at my side. The one who understood my need for happiness through sugar.

"So . . . I've started to change my life a little. I mean . . . after you left it was pretty ugly. Mom and Kenzie cried for months and months. I ate all of our favorite foods all the time because . . . well, that's what we always did, I guess. I felt like I lost my best friend when you died and I didn't really know how to—"

The words wobbled in my throat. Like a flow of magma, tears rushed to the surface of my eyes, making them feel like hot, stinging sandpaper. My next whisper came out rushed and choked.

"Why did we do that? Why did we eat so much? Why did you let me eat a meal-sized snack after school every day? Now I'm overweight and unhappy and you're dead. You didn't take care of your health, and now you're gone and Mom is lonely and depressed and McKenzie is getting married in five months and you're not here. You're not here!"

The vehemence of my own words caught me by surprise, so I sucked in a shaky breath to stop the intense feeling. I didn't like how betrayed I felt, or how wonderful it was to admit that even though he'd been my world, I was still angry that he hadn't taught me how to cope without sugar. It opened a dam that I hadn't even known existed deep inside my chest. The waters gushed out with every heavy thud of my heart.

"I guess . . . I guess I'm kind of mad at you. You didn't teach me to take care of myself. Mom always made me feel like looking beautiful was the most important part of being healthy. And now I'm finding people that say . . . that say I should eat healthy because it's the right thing to do. And you never taught me that. And now it's too late."

As final as the words felt when I said them, a flash of Megan's face in my eyes made it seem like I was wrong.

"Well . . . maybe my fate isn't sealed," I murmured, remembering how it felt to lose five pounds. I reached down, fingering the loose material around my legs. "Maybe now that I know more I can turn things around for me. I can be healthy. I can be happy, even. Maybe I'll even start liking carrot sticks."

A traitorous laugh, surprisingly bright and light in the sudden dark chasm that I'd found myself in, rippled through me. I reached out and traced his name with a finger and a deep longing in my heart.

"I guess I'm not really mad at you, Dad." Several tears slipped over my eyelid and slipped down my face. "I think I'm just sad. I'm so very sad for what both of us have missed out on so far."

"You can open your eyes, Lexie."

"I can't, Bitsy. Tell me what it says."

"You're the only person that is this dramatic about getting weighed, you know that?"

"I don't care. Tell me."

"What if I refuse?"

"Then you're a heartless taskmaster."

She sighed. I could picture her baby bangs dancing on top of her forehead. I had my eyes clenched shut, my hands fisted at my side, and was so nervous about what the scale would say that I had to pee— never mind that I'd insisted on tinkling before Bitsy weighed me.

"249. You lost three pounds."

My eyes flew open. "What?" I screeched. She smiled, though it didn't quite take away the rampant fatigue in her eyes.

"Congratulations! You are officially out of the 250's and well on your way to a healthier life. Just look at your pants. They're going to fall off soon."

I blinked and looked to the confirmation on the front of the scale. 249. An exhale of relief escaped me. I didn't maintain, and I didn't gain, and I was out of the 250's to never return. I suppressed the urge to fist pump, and wondered if I should text Megan to tell her the good news.

"Whew."

Bitsy had already scribbled it on her clipboard. She stepped back and motioned for me to exit the bathroom with all the finesse of a drill instructor.

"You broke through it and have been successful. You did good, Lexie."

I smiled. "I know."

"Now the most important thing is keeping it up." Her eyes narrowed in a strict warning. "Don't fall off the bandwagon now by celebrating with pie or something like that."

To my surprise, not even the pie sounded good to me. I grabbed my Nalgene of fresh ice water off the bathroom counter with a wide grin.

"Forget pie. Let's talk about working out!"

Chapter 27—You're Different

"Do you really want this internship, Lexie?"

My advisor, Miss Bliss, stared at me from over the rim of her horn-rimmed glasses. I hadn't known that people actually wore those kinds of things outside of Hollywood.

"Yes, Miss Bliss."

She shuffled a few papers in front of her, as if she could find the answer to my plea for help inside them somewhere.

"Then you're going to need to beef up your resume."

"I've been taking those free classes online on how to use Microsoft Word and Excel so I can put them on my resume—"

"That may help," she interrupted me with a pompous air. "But you need more. This is an extremely competitive internship. Winning it could guarantee you a slot right into the publishing business. That is what you want, isn't it?"

"Yes, Miss Bliss."

Miss Bliss wore a grayish blonde bouffant I thought I'd once seen Doris Day wear in the old romances that Mom and Kenzie loved. Complete with the jewelry dripping from her neck and the hot pink lipstick stains on her teeth, Miss Bliss lived the definition of *eternal spinster.*

"I've sent students to this internship before, and have never heard from them again, which is just what we want. It helps them disappear into the publishing industry in New York and pursue their dreams. But first you need to demonstrate that you have an exceptional talent and eye for words yourself."

My forehead ruffled. "How do I do that?"

"By winning a writing competition. Or two. Two would be great. Or one big one."

Writing wasn't new to me; I wanted to be an editor, after all. But writing for other people to read it? That didn't interest me. I wanted to be the person behind the scenes. The one that read the story, made it perfect, and enjoyed the secret feeling of knowing that another person's success had been aided by my expertise.

"I don't write for competitions."

She leveled a narrow eye on me. "Then you don't win competitive internships with publishing companies."

"I want to edit, Miss Bliss. Not write for other people. I'm not good in the spotlight. I don't like attention on me."

"Fine. But you can't be a good editor if you don't know good writing. No publishing company is going to hire an editor that hasn't proven her mettle somehow."

I opened my mouth to counter, but had no way to do so. She was right; proving that I knew the industry would help. Padding my resume with a few competitions, classes, and writing or editing conferences could help. Even get me a ticket out of my town and away from my mom.

"I see what you're saying," I admitted reluctantly. Miss Bliss licked her thumb and pulled a piece of paper from the pile in front of her.

"I took the liberty of printing off a few competitions that I think would be good for you to enter. Winning anything would be nice, but something bigger would be better. Enter as many as you can. We have four months until the application is due. Let's make the best of it."

She smiled with her smeared teeth in a self-congratulatory way, no doubt convinced she was the best advisor on the planet. I had to give her some credit; she was certainly more helpful—if not forceful—than I had expected.

"Thank you, Miss Bliss," I said, folding the paper up without looking at the list. "I'll get to work right away."

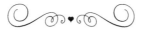

A long sigh escaped me later that night. I sat at my desk in my basement lair, the list of writing competitions unfurled in front of me and rested on my keyboard. Most of them were guaranteed to have thousands of entries. A few were local enough to only merit around one hundred. But still . . .

Lexie Greene did not share her writing.

With another sigh of uncertainty, I shoved the list of contests into my top drawer and leaned back in the chair. Rachelle sent me a text announcing she was on her way over to watch a movie, and I tried to mentally prepare myself to refuse the massive bag of buttery, salty popcorn delight I knew she'd bring with her.

The familiar little chime of a Facebook message broke through my reverie.

Are we both busy or something? Bradley asked. *I feel like we never really chat anymore.*

I smiled. We used to talk every night. But now I was busy doing . . . well . . . *life.* It was a new experience for me. One I wished I'd participated in more often.

We must be. Sometimes I feel like I never stop studying or working at the pub. What's going on with you?

He sent a sheepish smiley face with a blush. *I'm studying and deciding whether I want to switch my major to engineering . . . and feeling guilty because I still haven't read Frankenstein the way I promised.*

I laughed and glanced at the book on my desk. Neither had I.

Don't worry. I've been too busy also.

How's the diet going? I'm not doing too hot over here in the food department, but I've been working out every day.

My throat constricted. Although the ice had been broken with Bradley, I still felt uncomfortable talking with him about what food I did or didn't eat. That topic came far too close to my secret life of devil's food cake and oatmeal cream pies and skirted the edges of my less-than-perfect appearance.

Not so bad.

Still plan on outrunning me when I get there? ;)

"Uh . . ." I whispered shakily. "Only if you run 20 minute miles."

Obviously, I boasted, feeling obligated to keep up with the arrogance of it all. My hands shook as I responded. *I look forward to it.*

All right, tough girl. I need to get going. Later.

"HEY!" Rachelle's voice boomed from the top of the stairs. She sang in an exaggerated, horrific, opera impersonation. "I have arrived!"

She stumbled slowly down the stairs—girls like us just couldn't move gracefully while walking into gravity—in a long flowing gown and her hair done in a riot of curls.

"Let me guess," I drawled, glad to close Facebook and spin the chair to look at her. "You brought *Phantom of the Opera* to watch?

Are we going to have to rewind and watch "The Point of No Return" three times?"

She pulled a DVD from the depths of her ample cleavage. "Duh! What else are we going to watch on a Saturday night? The only man I want to spend *any* weekend with is Gerard Butler. And yes. We'll watch it as many times as needed."

I stood up to take the movie, but a funny look crossed Rachelle's face and stopped me. She stared at me, appearing puzzled.

"What?" I asked self-consciously. "Do I have something on my face?"

"No, it's just that . . . you're different."

"Different?"

Her expression fell. "Your face looks . . . thinner."

I sucked in a breath and tried to hide my excitement with a careless facade. "Oh?"

"Yeah. Are you still doing that salad thing?"

"Sure. It's kind of become a habit."

She gestured to my clothes in a helpless way. "I haven't seen that shirt before."

I glanced down to find an old concert t-shirt that Kenzie had brought me when she went to a Backstreet Boys show with Mom. It was the largest size available and I'd had it for years. Dad and I had stayed behind to watch a football game from the safety of our couches because neither of us liked crowds.

"I found it in my drawer."

Rachelle blinked, staring at me in a rare moment of vulnerability. "You aren't going to change on me, are you? You aren't going to be too good for me if I'm not skinny?"

My expression softened. "What are you talking about? You're my best friend. You always will be. Jean size doesn't apply."

She scrutinized me with extreme attention. Apparently finding my response agreeable, she bounced over to the ratty old couch with a giant bag of popcorn in tow.

"Great! Let's get started. My future husband awaits!"

Chapter 28—Farewell DDP

The next week I shuffled out of Bitsy's bathroom with a smug sense of triumph. Two more pounds down, which brought my total to twelve pounds in five weeks. I still had dreams of creamsicles dancing through my brain at night, but at least the daydreams had stopped plaguing me.

Mira waited for me on the couch in one of her bright muumuus. She had also lost more weight, if the dreamy look in her eyes meant anything. Although, true to Bitsy's word, none of us exchanged weight loss numbers.

"Where are the boys?" I asked as I sat down, noticing for the first time that they hadn't come. The couch creaked beneath me, a constant reminder that though I'd come a long way, I still had a ways to go.

"Yeah," Mira piped up, echoing my surprise. "Where are they?"

All three of us stared across Bitsy's living room to the empty couch where the two men normally sat. One of them hadn't come the week before, and the other had been ten minutes late.

"They've quit," Bitsy declared, lips pursed. The sound of giggles and shrieks floated from the back room where her little girls played. "Both of them called me this week and said they didn't have time for it anymore."

The thought deflated me almost as much as stepping on the scale again. Seriously? Why would they quit? Thoughts of doughnuts and blueberry muffin tops floated through my mind and I understood.

Dieting sucked.

"It's all right," Bitsy declared, rallying admirably. "We don't need them to lose weight. We still have each other, and that's all we need. Besides, you can lose weight on your own. It's just harder. So now it will be the three girls standing strong together. Because isn't that what always happens anyway?"

"Hear, hear!" Mira called, raising a chubby fist in the sky. She'd just had her nails done, so they glowed a bright hot pink. "The *Health and Happiness Society* continues on—"

"—With a lesson about the dangers of drinking diet pop," Bitsy said, picking up right where Mira left off. I scowled when she handed me a paper with the words *Diet Soda: Worse than Regular?*

"Whoa, Bits," I said, holding up a hand. "This is going too far. Caffeine is the only thing that gets me through the day. I'd fall asleep in my classes because I'm so tired from working out every morning without Diet Dr Pepper."

"You'd feel better without any at all," she insisted, perching on the edge of a chair across from us. "The caffeine is what's making you tired, not the exercise. It gives you energy, sure, but then drops you like a rock so you need more. It's all a conspiracy."

I opened my mouth to protest, but she stopped me.

"Let's just talk about the ingredients in a randomly selected diet pop on the market: *Diet Dr Pepper.*"

I glared at her. Randomly selected my—

"I'll read first," she said.

Like me, Mira looked a bit pale. She'd eventually shucked her Pepsi addiction, but had switched her tune to Diet. Though she wouldn't admit it, I knew she must have consumed at least six a day to replace the sugary sweetness of Pepsi. Although Bitsy wouldn't believe me, the caffeine really did take away some of my cravings for food. That, or it just gave me a different flavor so I felt like I was eating.

"Diet Dr Pepper is sweetened with aspartame, which has been linked with cancer," Bitsy began matter-of-factly. "There's also sodium benzoate, which is a derivative of petroleum or coal tar . . . "

Bitsy droned on and on, effectively tightening the very few muscles I had in my stomach and making me sicker. Before last week I wouldn't have really cared: Diet Dr Pepper was going to help me get hot for Bradley. I'd deal with the consequences later. But now, after meeting Megan, after having an epiphany, after realizing that weight loss wasn't just supposed to be about my swimsuit size, I couldn't ignore it.

This was about health just as much as it was about size, wasn't it? Well, it was supposed to be. Although most days I wasn't really sure I bought into that whole spiel.

I needed to give up Diet Dr Pepper.

The thought of not drinking my favorite cold, slightly sweet and tangy beverage made my throat tighten. I always looked forward to my DDP fix. Hadn't I given up enough already? Would dieting take away all the things that I enjoyed?

"Well Lexie?" Bitsy asked, breaking into my depressing train of thought. "What do you think? Will you commit to giving it up for just one week? Then we can reevaluate next week and see how differently you feel?"

I sighed. It wasn't like I could avoid it anymore.

"Yes."

Mira and I shared a frightened look. This wasn't going to be a pretty week. I tried to cheer myself up with the reminder that I had already lost twelve pounds and putting aside diet pop could help me lose some more. Time ticked down with every day that passed. My meeting with Bradley was less than four months away now. Every single day had to count.

"Wonderful!" Bitsy cried. "I know it will be hard, but trust me, it's worth it. I had to give up Mountain Dew years ago, and though I went through withdrawals at first, now I'd never go back. Your body, and your kidneys, will thank you."

Chapter 29—Zumba

By Saturday night I was a hot, desperate mess of Diet Dr Pepper withdrawal.

Giving up that sweet, magic elixir cold turkey sent my body into a strange hole. I had a new sympathy for Alice in Wonderland. My workouts lagged. My motivation to diet suffered. I went over my calories every day by at least three hundred. The bland taste of water all but revolted me.

To add insult to injury, I still hadn't thought of a good entry to write so I could submit to one of the competitions Miss Bliss wanted me to win for the editing internship. Two of them were big. Those, I figured, I had to at least try.

Except nothing about the week after the weigh-in was going well.

Mira sent me a text that she had a migraine Saturday morning and wouldn't be able to work out. I stayed in bed, staring at the glow-in-the-dark stars on my ceiling and listening to the howling blizzard outside with a scowl. Not even the thought of possibly running into Megan made me want to get up. In fact, I didn't want to see anyone right then that wasn't bearing an ice-cold can of DDP. When it's just cold enough to be slushy but not frozen and tasted like—

"Lex?"

A light tap on my bedroom door followed Kenzie's inquiry. She hadn't walked down the stairs and into my basement lair for months.

"Yeah?"

"Are you busy?"

I pushed the covers off, slipped out of bed, and pulled the door open. Lithe, beautiful Kenzie—who surely hadn't ever eaten an entire box of cosmic brownies on her own—stood in a pair of tight black yoga pants and a fitted tank top, never mind the horrid weather swirling outside. She had the audacity to smile.

"Good morning!" she chirped.

"What do you want, Kenz?"

She bit her bottom lip and fidgeted with the bottom of her tank top. "I . . . uh . . . had a question."

"Ok."

"Will you work out with me today?"

"What?"

"It's just that I've noticed you're counting calories and working out every morning with Mira at the gym. You're looking really good too. We've never really exercised together before because, well, you've never exercised before, so I thought it might be fun if we have some sister bonding time and . . . you know . . . work out together."

She said it in a frantic rush, as if she were afraid I'd say no if she didn't talk 100 miles per hour. I blinked. Except for having dinner together when Dad was alive, we hadn't ever really done much *sister bonding* time. I wondered if this had something to do with the fact that she'd be moving away this summer after she got married. She wouldn't be flittering around the house, singing the latest Kelly Clarkson song under her breath or making me feel inferior because of her tiny little waist.

The thought made me a little sad.

"Kenzie, you'd eat me alive in a workout. I can barely wog."

She grinned and held up a flyer that I hadn't seen in her hands. Big black letters sprawled across the top.

ZUMBA DANCE PARTY.

"That's why we're going to Zumba."

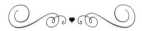

I didn't believe Kenzie's reassurances that *you'll just love it, Lexie. It's working out and being sexy at the same time,* so I stressed the whole way to the gym.

Dance in front of others? To music? What would they think when my stomach jiggled? What if they laughed because I wasn't sexy? Didn't they have mirrors so I'd see my cottage cheese fleshy arms if I lifted them above my shoulders?

"Oh good," Kenzie said when we walked into the room. "Stephanie is teaching it today. She's fabulous."

I stepped into the room and tried to keep my mouth from falling to the floor. While I'd heard of Zumba before, I didn't realize it was popular. In fact, lots of woman did Zumba.

And lots of them were my size.

Kenzie giggled. "See?" she asked, seeing the look on my face. "I told you! It's like a safe girl haven. Guys hardly ever come. Besides, no one will be looking at you. They'll just be watching Stephanie or themselves."

She stashed her car keys and coat in a cubby on the wall, waving to a few people in the crowd. I hadn't even known Kenzie came to things like this, let alone knew people there.

"So what do I do?" I asked, trailing right behind her, feeling a bit lost. The big crowd meant I could hide in the back and avoid the awkward confrontation-of-self with the mirrors.

"Just follow whatever Stephanie does. She's that girl at the front with the microphone."

"The one with a six-pack and toned arms that would make Jennifer Aniston weep?"

Kenzie laughed. "Yes, that one."

Despite the anonymity of the milling crowd, I still felt nervous while glancing over the fifty or so women present. Some of them, like me, didn't make eye contact with anyone else and still managed to studiously avoid looking at themselves in the mirror.

To my delight, the lights flipped off moments later. A disco ball descended from the ceiling, and the Jennifer-Aniston-Wannabe Stephanie hopped onto a platform at the top of the room.

"WHO'S READY FOR ZUMBA?" she cried. I already wanted to hate her but couldn't because she was one of those attractive people you couldn't hate. Her enthusiasm was infectious. A little buzz of excitement rippled through me. Maybe this could be fun.

A wild cheer rang through the crowd just as an upbeat song blasted through the speakers. I tried not to feel like I was in a rave, but couldn't help but feel fascinated by the excitement.

And not one of those women looked at me.

I relaxed a little and turned my attention to Stephanie.

"We've got a new routine, new songs, and a great butt blaster workout planned for today. So let's start with a warm-up!"

Seconds later I joined the world of Zumba.

I squatted, hopped, shook my hips, slid, twirled, waved my hands, and danced in combinations that I'd never before dreamed. I sweated, laughed, panted, and cursed under my breath when we held a squat for thirty seconds. Under the cover of the dark room and so many women just like me, I stopped caring about what others might be thinking, or whether my body moved in ugly ways underneath my too-loose t-shirt.

After a while, I just enjoyed the music and danced.

"Here," Kenzie said, throwing a towel at me at the end. She grinned, her neck glistening with sweat. "Great, isn't it?"

"Yeah. It wasn't so bad."

"You should buy a heart rate monitor and see how many calories you burn. It's a better workout than the elliptical I bet."

I couldn't argue with that. Sweat had accumulated underneath my nose, something I didn't even know could happen during a workout.

"How often do you come?" I asked. "I'd . . . I'd like to do this again. Maybe a couple times?"

We shared a silent moment of sisterhood, something that I couldn't recall ever happening before unless it was bonding over a shared banana split when I was ten.

Kenzie's smile widened. "I'd love that. I come three times a week to Stephanie's classes in the evening."

The idea perked me up. I could still work out with Mira in the mornings and add an extra workout in a few times a week to lose even more weight.

"Come on," Kenzie said, grabbing her coat. "Let's go buy a healthy smoothie or something. There's a new mango flavor that I'm just dying to try."

Chapter 30—The Dreaded Plateau

"You're awfully cheery tonight," Mira observed the next Wednesday evening, eyeing me askance as she climbed out of her car. "Since when did you look forward to coming to Bitsy's house?"

A light snow crunched beneath my feet as I walked toward the front door. Mira held onto the fence for balance.

"Since I started Zumba with Kenzie. I've been working out twice a day. It's so much fun that I go every night before dinner."

Mira perked up. "Really? That's wonderful!"

Mira didn't get all weird or defensive when other people showed motivation or weight loss, the way I would have. She just beamed at me like a proud Mama. It was my favorite thing about her.

"This weigh-in is going to rock, Mira! I can feel it. I'm thinking I've lost at least five pounds, maybe six."

She tugged at my loose size eighteen pants. I wore them as a trophy. Having them so baggy I couldn't feel the material on my legs made me feel like a champion. Mira rang the doorbell, and the familiar shrieks of two little girls hopping by the window and into their back bedroom followed. Bitsy opened the door looking a bit haggard. She wore her workout clothes as usual, but appeared so tired that I thought we might have woken her up.

"Come on in," she said with a tight smile, swinging the door open and motioning inside. "Please excuse my mess. It's been a long day."

Bitsy's *mess* consisted of a few dirty dishes stacked next to the sink in the kitchen, a quiet rerun of *Mickey Mouse Clubhouse* playing on the TV, and a few toys on the floor. The rest of her house looked as in-place as usual. Her daughters giggled and laughed from the back room before slamming the door closed.

"You all right, Bits?" Mira asked, her eyebrows furrowing. "You seem . . . tired."

Bitsy rubbed her eyes and ran a hand over her face. "It's been a long day."

Mira's questioning gaze deepened into one of greater understanding. "Problems with the girls?"

"My ex is giving me trouble over child support again."

They had a silent exchange, and Mira's nostrils flared with rage. Something in my chest lurched for Bitsy. Her ex? My eyes quickly sped around the room to all the pictures. A dark-haired man lingered in a couple. I'd never met or seen any man around the house before, and had just assumed she was still married. Bitsy must have seen the confusion in my eyes because she spoke up before I could ask.

"We divorced two years ago when he cheated on me with his secretary. I keep the pictures of him up for the girls, who adore him, but don't get to see him much these days. It's all they really have."

"He's a prig," Mira stated. "An ugly, ugly man hiding behind a pretty face. I can say that because I've met him."

A semblance of a smile appeared in Bitsy's eyes, but disappeared quickly. "Yes, a prig. Let's not talk about him anymore. Let's get started with the meeting."

She motioned for me to sit down, and she and Mira walked down the hall to the scale. Instead of sitting, I walked up to the pictures and studied them. Bitsy's husband had been an extremely attractive man. Tall, lean, muscular, with a bright smile and dark hair. But what did that matter if he had the personality of a lech? I thought of Bradley, whom I hadn't spoken with in almost two days now, and wondered if maybe I was just being fooled by a pair of light eyes. Apparently being attractive wasn't the most important thing.

Mira and Bitsy shuffled back out of the bathroom a few minutes later. Mira's eyes lit up.

"A wonderful weigh-in is right!" she declared, grinning. Bitsy must have reminded her of the strict no-numbers policy, for Mira didn't elaborate anymore. But I caught her enthusiasm and remembered my initial excitement.

This was going to be the best weigh-in *ever.*

With light feet I followed Bitsy back to the pastel room of terror. Now that I looked at it, however, it didn't seem so bad. The baby blue was a bit overdone, but it was a nice bathroom.

"All right," Bitsy said, clipboard in hand, defenses firmly in place again behind her steely eyes. "Let's see how well you've done this week."

"It's going to be awesome," I declared, stepping out of my shoes and peeling my jacket off. "I've been working out twice a day with my sister, who is actually pretty cool it turns out. My calories have been right on and—"

My heart stuttered to a stop.

247.

"Bitsy," I whispered. "Does the scale say the same number it said last week?"

Her forehead crinkled. "Oh, yes," she said in surprise. "It does."

Dreams of reaching 240 disintegrated in my hands like melting flakes of snow. "How?" I whispered, feeling hoarse. "How can that be?"

She wrote the number down and shrugged. "Probably just a plateau. It happens sometimes."

"What's a plateau?" I cried, whirling around to face her and nearly falling off the scale.

"It just means you've hit a spot where your numbers aren't going down. Maybe your increased workouts caused it. Give it time. You'll work through. Maybe try eating back some of the calories that you burn. You don't want to under eat because your body still needs calories to function and to burn."

My mouth bobbed up and down. I hadn't been this surprised at a number since the scale first flashed the ugly truth of *259* on my first weigh-in. I sank to the toilet feeling wobbly.

"But I've felt so good this week!" I cried. "I've worked so hard. I've tracked everything. I drank more water than a fish. I didn't even eat a Cinnabon when Rachelle offered to buy one for me! It's not fair!"

Bitsy pressed her lips together. "Lots of things in life aren't fair, Lex. You just have to keep going."

I pulled in a breath. In the aftermath of all her very real problems, I felt ashamed reacting to my simple little issue.

She pointed her pen at me. "Don't let this derail you. I've had plateaus that have lasted for three weeks. You'll work through it eventually, trust me."

"Three weeks?" I gasped. "I don't have three weeks to waste on a plateau!"

"Because you're still determined to work out for that guy?"

"Uh, no. I just . . . I just have a life to live and it won't be a very long one if I keep carrying all this weight around."

Bitsy rolled her eyes. "Right. Come on, let's go. We'll discuss plateaus out here with Mira. I think you'll feel better once you realize how common they are."

"I'd rather burn the scale," I muttered, sliding my shoes back on with a low growl of frustration. Images of my missed Cinnabon danced through my brain. A good dollop of frosting would really hit the spot. I might as well have eaten the pastry for all that depriving myself got me.

"I'll start the fire," Bitsy offered, flicking the light off. "We'll use my old wedding certificate as kindling."

Chapter 31—Plate o' Bacon

I stood immobile on the treadmill Thursday morning after my failed weigh-in.

The numbers flashed a bright, enticing green. I waited to see if they'd communicate the secret to weight loss. *Run at 5.0 for 100 hours, and you'll be skinny and only weigh 120 pounds.*

Oh, the dream.

The endless stream of pointless green words continued to scroll across the screen in a dull advertisement. Nope. No such secrets spilled. No matter what lies I told myself about working out, I couldn't find any motivation. What was the point of working so hard if the scale didn't change?

"Plateaus," I said bitterly. "As if dieting wasn't difficult enough."

"Hey." Megan approached from the side, her brown braid swinging from the back of her head. "I wondered if I'd see you this morning. Uh oh. What's wrong?" She wore a pair of fingerless gloves and her usual black yoga pants. I turned away to hide my scowl. At this rate, I'd never fit into yoga pants. Never be able to work out with Bradley without looking like a fool.

"Nothing," I mumbled. "Just don't want to be here."

She agreed with a quiet little snort, looking over her shoulder to where her friend awaited at the racks. "Me either. I'm facing some gnarly overhead squats today. I love to hate them."

I glanced over at her in a last push of desperation. There was no one else to talk to about my problem that I felt could *maybe* understand; although, I doubted a girl like Megan had ever been my size. She wasn't supermodel skinny, but I'd still kill to have a toned body like her.

"Megan, have you ever tried to lose weight?"

"Of course. I was the heaviest kid in elementary school when I grew up. Junior high too. I started figuring it out in high school when I picked up running with my best friend." Her eyes narrowed. "Why?"

"I just . . . it sucks, right? Is it supposed to be hard and discouraging and endless and frustrating and up and down?"

Her expression softened.

"Yeah, it does suck. It sucks a lot. But nothing great in life is ever easy, right?"

"It's pretty easy to eat a plate of bacon and I feel like that's pretty great."

To my surprise, she laughed.

"But seriously! What's the point?" I asked, throwing my hands in the air. "Why am I working so hard if the scale isn't going to show it? I literally worked my butt off at Zumba, and in the mornings last week, but I didn't lose a single pound. I counted calories to the bite. I drank so much water I was floating. What more can I do?"

She leaned against the empty treadmill bars behind me, a little smirk of amusement on her face.

"First of all: Why are you working for the scale?" she asked.

"What?"

I stared at her in confusion. She shrugged. "What does the scale have to do with anything?"

"Uh . . . everything."

"The scale doesn't mean anything."

"I . . . I don't understand."

"Lex, the scale is just a number. It doesn't reflect health. You've been working on weight machines right?"

"Yeah."

"Muscles weighs more than fat. So you're getting stronger, but smaller."

My eyes popped open. "Seriously?"

"Serious. What if you're bloated? The scale will go up. What if you're muscular? The scale will say you're too heavy, but you might be in great shape. Screw the scale. Throw it away. It's worthless."

If I hadn't already been holding onto the handrails, I would have fallen. Megan had a habit of throwing curveballs into all my opinions on life and health.

The scale was the symbol of weight loss and hotness, right?

"Throw away the scale?" I repeated dumbly. "But that's insane. How will I know if I've made any progress?"

She straightened and motioned toward my pants with a tilt of her head. "How are your clothes fitting?"

"Loose."

"How do you feel after a workout?"

"Hungry."

She laughed again, and I cracked my first smile for the day. My stomach growled in testament.

"Okay, granted, I feel hungry after working out too. But do you feel anything else?"

"Of course. I feel good after I work out. Happy, even."

She met my gaze straight on. "And how do you feel every morning when you wake up now compared to a couple months ago when you first started getting healthier?"

I paused to think it over, because the intent look in her eyes told me this wasn't something to take lightly. I thought of my basement lair, of the secret stash of food I used to have in my closet, but didn't anymore. I thought of Zumba with Kenzie and the light, fresh taste of a healthy, non-sugary smoothie. My last thought culminated on the realization that I hadn't even logged onto Facebook the past two days because I'd been too busy.

That had never happened before now. Facebook—or perhaps it had just been Bradley—was all that I had looked forward to every day. Now I had new friends and new goals.

"I feel great," I concluded with a sheepish smile. "I feel . . . alive."

Megan smiled.

"Yeah," she said. "And you look alive. That's what getting healthy is about. Getting healthy is more up here than anywhere else." She tapped on the side of her head. "It's not just counting calories. I eat clean because it's good for my body. But I exercise because it's how I feel good about myself. I prove I can do hard things, and I feel like a boss."

Megan was so *different*. Although I couldn't deny that watching the numbers tick down on the scale was euphoric, maybe even addicting, Megan had a light in her eyes and a sense of confidence that I had never even hoped for. I didn't exactly understand how, but I had the vague impression that her courage had something to do with her strange philosophies on life and exercise.

"I never thought of the problem being in my head," I said, leaning against the treadmill arms. "I always thought it was in my tree-trunk sized legs."

Megan tilted her head back and laughed again.

"Just let it go, Lex. Forget the scale. Don't work out so that the numbers go down, because the numbers are fickle. Do it because it makes you happy and because it's the right thing to do for your body. The pounds will melt off, and in the meantime, you'll find yourself."

Bradley: *Hey Lex! How are things going?*

Lexie: *Good! I just got back from the gym.*

Bradley: *Nice. Good workout?*

Lexie: *Yeah. Intervals on the treadmill and a few weight machines. Nothing crazy. I talked with my friend Megan for a while too. It was . . . enlightening.*

Bradley: *Oh?*

Lexie: *Yeah. She just always gives me something to think about.*

Bradley: *Here's something else to think about. I'm almost done with reading Frankenstein. (Be impressed.)*

Lexie: *I am!*

Bradley: *So I was thinking that we could discuss it next weekend? I'm busy this weekend with a few things, but I'd love to talk about it next week.*

Lexie: *Sure. I'm free.*

Bradley: *Awesome. Because I think it would be awesome to video chat. What do you say?*

Chapter 32—Coming Around

"Why did I say yes? WHY? I don't want to video chat with Bradley! That's . . . it's insane."

I raked my nails down the side of my face and hung my head in resignation. No matter how much I beat myself up over it now, it didn't matter. In three days, I was going to video chat with the supposed love of my life and I still had chubby-girl cheeks. Surely he'd close the connection, or recoil, or suddenly become too busy to talk.

"WHY?"

To make matters worse, it was Wednesday. Weigh-in day. I pushed away the salad with balsamic vinaigrette and dropped my head onto my folded arms. Rachelle, completely apathetic to my internal torment, took another bite of cheese pizza.

"Because you secretly want to see him," she said. "I mean really. He's beautiful, right? I've seen the Facebook pictures. Mostly just his face and shoulders though. Have you noticed that? Not that it matters. He looks totally ripped."

I groaned from the cave my arms made. "I know! And I look . . . totally *not* ripped. He should be dating someone like Megan."

Rachelle quirked an eyebrow. "Who is Megan?"

"A friend from the gym."

Her eyes widened. "You make friends at the gym? Seriously? You talk to people there? I wouldn't even make eye contact. Then again, I've never gone to a gym . . ."

"Just one friend. Can we focus on Bradley and my upcoming embarrassment?"

Rachelle dropped her pizza and leaned forward to stare at me over the table. She wore no costume today, opting for a simple pair of jeans, a t-shirt, and her hair in two braided pigtails. Without makeup, she had a sweet, almost girlish expression. I couldn't help but wonder what had prompted this strange turn of normalcy.

"Lexie, get over it," she said. "You're awesome. And if he can't see that—which obviously he has already because he's always contacting you and trying to be friends despite how creepy Facebook is—then he wouldn't be worth it." Her expression drooped a little. "At least you have a Bradley, you know? It gives you someone to at least dream about in the lonely nights."

"Are you lonely?" I asked.

Rachelle, who had always proclaimed herself proud of being overweight, who had openly asked men on dates while dressed like Rainbow Brite, suddenly looked like an uncertain little girl.

All traces of vulnerability disappeared with a saucy little scoff. "No. Of course not. I don't *need* a man, I just like having them around when it suits my purposes, the bloody apes. But I can see that you have been, especially since your dad died. Bradley gives you a spark of hope."

Despite her smooth cover, something lingered in her expression that I couldn't read. I turned away, not sure what I could say, or should say, to make it better. Maybe I couldn't.

I'm not skinny enough for a great guy like Bradley, I almost said, but stopped myself. Megan and Bitsy ran through my mind. Had Bitsy been *skinny enough* for her husband? What about the many boyfriends that had dumped Megan—whom I thought was just shy of perfect? Had she been *skinny enough* for them? What if I did all this work for nothing?

Not skinny enough?

I'd had the thought at least a thousand times before, but it rang differently tonight. It seemed wrong, although I didn't completely understand why.

What if, in the end, weight didn't really matter?

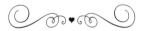

Bitsy met Mira and I at the door that night with a tense smile. Her house—as immaculate as ever—lay in unusually pristine, quiet condition. The silence was the first thing I noticed when I stepped inside.

"Where are your girls?" Mira asked. Bitsy's lips tightened.

"With their father. He's in town for the week and took them out to dinner tonight."

Ah. Tension.

Mira and I shuffled quietly in, settling in our usual spots on the couch. I'd come in the same thing I wore every week now. Flip-flops, a pair of scrub pants weighing only a few ounces, and an old t-shirt. Bitsy sent me an imploring look as she shut the door behind us.

"I think it's time for someone to get a new shirt," she said, eyeing the long, swaying folds of the one I wore. Granted, it fit me like one of Mira's muumuus. But at least it hid my love handles and my oddly shaped bum.

"Time to go shopping!" Mira cried, clapping. "I love shopping. Your mother would be ecstatic if we got you a new wardrobe!"

"Ready to start?" Bitsy asked, pulling her clipboard off a bookshelf. Her eyes drilled right into mine. "Let's go weigh in."

I opened my sweaty palm and pressed it against my pants. Here it was. The confrontation I'd been dreading almost as much as video chatting with Bradley in a couple of days.

"Uh . . . can I talk to you about that?"

Bitsy stopped mid-stride. Mira's head whipped round to face me.

"What's up?" Bitsy drawled.

A thick lump sat in my throat; I swallowed it back. "I . . . uh . . . I'm thinking about scaling back on weighing in."

"Scaling back?"

"To just once a month."

Both Mira and Bitsy stared at me in shock. "But why?" Mira asked incredulously. "How else are you going to lose weight?"

"Well I'll still lose weight, I'll just change my focus," I stammered uncertainly, suddenly fearing that I hadn't made the right decision after all. "I spoke with a friend last week, and I've been thinking about the scale ever since. I want to . . . I want to try losing weight for the right reasons. I don't mean that the scale is a *bad* reason, I just mean that it's become the main reason for me. Except for, well . . . anyway . . ."

The edges of Bitsy's lips curled up ever-so-slightly, enough to send a flutter of nervous energy through my chest. Was that approval?

Did Bitsy actually agree with me?

"And what is the right reason?" she asked with the clipped, direct tone of a mother. She held the clipboard against her chest. "Does the right reason involve a boy?"

I bit my bottom lip.

"It used to involve a boy. And looking hot for him when we met," I admitted, a hot flush of blood rising to my cheeks. "But now I'm wondering if looking hot is really enough. I mean . . . boys dump Megan all the time, and my parents weren't always happy together, and your husband is a douche bag. So . . ." I wasn't entirely sure how to end my thoughts in a way that wasn't the question: *What if losing weight for a boy isn't the point of all this? What if there's more?*

"Interesting," Bitsy murmured with a side-glance at Mira, who was beaming.

"I want to weigh in just once a month because I still want to see progress. I'll still track calories and come and work out every morning, I just want to see if removing the scale helps me focus better."

To my chagrin, Mira started to clap.

"I told you, Bits!" she called, eyes shining. "She'd come through. We knew she'd come through eventually!"

Bitsy smiled, and this time, there was no sign of uneasiness or tension. It lit up her face, making her appear young for a moment.

"Sounds like a good plan, Lexie."

"Just because you're breaking free from the scale doesn't mean I am," Mira called, using her fists to shove off the couch. "Let's go, Bits. You and I are still weighing in every week for a while. I need something to keep me on track and honest. I don't have a cute boy to do that for me."

She winked and the two of them disappeared into the hallway. Stunned that it had gone so well, I leaned back against the couch and smiled. Whether or not getting rid of the scale was the right decision, I felt good about it.

What an encouraging feeling.

Chapter 33—Just a Guy

I stared at my computer screen with the uncomfortable feeling of having just eaten a bowl of lava.

"Okay," I said through a soothing exhale. "Just relax. It's a video chat. Not a big deal. I'm ready. At least, I *better* be ready."

I'd only been puttering around my basement for the last two hours trying to straighten my hair and remember how to apply mascara.

Makeup? I thought, looking at the mirror next to my computer. *Check.* Although, admittedly, I hadn't worn makeup since before Dad died, so I kept it simple at foundation and mascara. The maturing effect startled me. While I still wasn't sure that I'd lost much weight in my face—I could never tell—Mira and Megan had reassured me that I had.

Outfit? A quick glance down confirmed that I hadn't forgotten to put on a new shirt. Mira had surprised me with it that morning at the gym just for this occasion.

"The color will make your eyes pop," she had reassured me. "Sometimes a new shirt is all you need to feel like a rock star."

The shirt, which was an XL, was smaller than any t-shirt I'd worn since high school. Okay, maybe even junior high.

I couldn't get over the miracle of it how it fit. A small boost of confidence made it seem like letting Bradley see my face might not be a total disaster. I completed the outfit with a pair of sweatpants and fuzzy bunny slippers. No reason to be *totally* uncomfortable. He wouldn't see below the neck anyway.

Door locked, I thought, glancing to the top of the stairs. No one would accidentally interrupt the most fateful call of my life.

"All set."

I was just about to check my phone for the billionth time when a familiar bell rang through my computer speakers. My blood froze. My heart stilled. I stared dumbly at the notification on my screen.

Incoming video call.

136

"Okay," I whispered again, smoothing my hair back one more time. "Okay. Okay. Okay. Okay. Okay."

But my hand remained. The computer continued to ring, echoing in long waves. I couldn't do it. Bradley, the love of my life, the only boy that had ever paid attention to me, waited on the other side of that call.

What if I disappointed him?

What if he didn't like me?

What if all my dreams shattered tonight?

On and on rang the video call.

A voice deep inside, one that I barely recognized as my own, rose through the layers of doubt. *What if I keep doing what I was doing and never take a chance? Then I'll never know.*

I reached forward and clicked "accept."

The connection was black for a second, although I could see myself in a small box in the corner, blinking. The lights in my lair were dim, but not too dim, so he could see my face but I wasn't blinding him with my pale winter skin. I'd tested it far too many times.

"Lexie? You there?"

A familiar face floated on the screen, distorted at first by the new connection, and then settled into an attractive smile. My heart skipped, making me breathless. He had a head of haphazard brown curls, giving his face a fuller, younger look. His hazel eyes, as smooth as pond water, were wide and thick with lashes.

"Bradley," I said, hoping it didn't sound as strangled as it felt. "Hey! How are you?"

"Oh, man!" He breathed a sigh of relief. "I'm so glad it worked! I've been worried all day that we'd have a bad connection or something." He grinned in a crooked boyish way that I had only seen in pictures. "Talking on the phone with a beautiful girl just isn't the same as seeing her face to face."

"No, it's not," I agreed weakly. The bowl of magma in my stomach churned. Did he just call me beautiful? Did he mean it? What if he was just flirtatious?

"Hey! I didn't know your eyes were green." He leaned toward the computer, eyes squinted, giving me a perfect shot of full lips and a soft face just touched with a sheen of stubble. "Are your eyes green?"

I laughed, feeling a bit self-conscious. "Yes. They always have been."

"Ah, yes. You got me there. You don't have very many pictures on Facebook, so I guess I never noticed. So hey, how was your day? Anything exciting happen? What's going on with that internship application? Talk to me about it."

I'd written a list of topics and taped it to the side of my monitor just in case we ran out, or didn't know where to start, but realized I likely wouldn't need them. Bradley had already started to put me at ease.

My heart fluttered again. *Who cares about an internship? Let's talk about falling in love with you.*

"It's . . . my internship application is . . . slow."

"Slow?"

"Yeah. My advisor wants me to write a bunch of stories for a couple of competitions. She thinks if my writing can win some awards, it will help pad my resume, show that I know what I'm doing."

He listened with genuine interest. "And how is writing going?"

I grimaced. "I'm stuck. I can't think of anything to write. I've tried every day for the past couple of weeks but . . . nothing."

He tutted under his breath as if he faced this kind of problem every day. "Ah. Not inspired?"

"Apparently not!" I replied through a laugh, trying my hardest not to look at the little box in the corner that betrayed my every movement. Was my laugh too high-pitched? Was my hair okay?

His expression sobered into one of real curiosity. He leaned forward, giving me a full view of his face and hiding a pair of shoulders that looked thick and strong beneath a simple white t-shirt. "Why aren't you inspired?" he asked. "There has to be a reason. Let's get to the bottom of it. Why do you want this internship?"

"You really want to do this?"

"Of course. I want to help you figure it out."

"O-okay. Well, I want to be an editor. The girl behind the scenes, you know? I don't want attention and spotlight."

He rolled his eyes. "It's a contest or two, Lex. Not a marriage proposal."

He said it so smooth, so easy, as if we'd been friends for our whole lives, that I felt the tense muscles in my shoulders ease back.

"Yeah, but it's still, you know. Personal."

"Writing?"

"Yes."

"Does personal scare you?" he asked.

"Sometimes."

He smiled. "Me too. But you have to do it to get what you want right? So maybe you're just not writing the right stuff. Let's brainstorm a few ideas. I think you should write a story about unicorns."

I tilted my head back and laughed. *This* was the slightly-dorky-but-endearing Bradley I'd known from Facebook and all our late night chats.

"Unicorns? Really?"

"Oh definitely. Unicorns that fart rainbows. What judge would turn that story down? None. I guarantee it." He held his hands up in surrender. "Just sayin'."

We tossed story ideas back and forth, giggling like school kids, until he stopped and said, "Hey, why don't you write about your dad's death?"

I reared back in surprise. "My dad?"

"You feel strongly about it, right? No doubt it would be some of your best writing. Maybe it would be a good outlet for you."

A knot had taken over my chest, effectively cutting off my ability to breathe or speak. Write about Dad? Write about how horrible those days were, how terrifyingly slow and fast and bleak? Putting words to Dad's death had never once crossed my mind. Wouldn't it resurrect all that pain?

All that pain you kept quiet by eating it back into submission? whispered my conscience, which had normally been silenced by my body-guard Little Debbie.

"Maybe," I managed to squeak out. "I'll . . . I'll think about it."

"The real question is this: Where are we going to eat on our first official date? Because food is kind of a big deal for a guy like me." He leaned back in his chair and stretched his arms over his head in a lazy, feline gesture.

His beautiful, muscular arms.

The transition in conversation, so well placed and easily executed, couldn't have been accidental. I had no doubt he'd done it because he'd noticed my discomfort. It made the downward spiral of my heart even stronger. I was falling so fast I expected to reach out and feel wind on my palm.

"Food?" I repeated, pulling words out of the back of my mind to cover how distracting I found his biceps. "Well, that's easy. We're going to a lot of restaurants."

He stopped stretching and lifted an eyebrow. "Oh?"

"Y-yeah," I said, forcing my voice to gain confidence. The vague idea grew on me. "Local restaurants, not chains. I know all the good food on the menus, trust me. We'll do an appetizer at the pub where I work, and you know, go out from there. My friend Megan showed me this great tiki hut place that serves the best smoothies and . . . what?"

His boyish grin had grown. He leaned forward again, arms folded, and leaned on them. It put his face closer to the camera, giving me an even better view of the flecks of gold in his eyes.

"See Lex? This is why I like you. You're different."

"Different?"

"Yeah. Different. You love the book *Frankenstein,* which is kind of a trip, by the way, but we'll talk about that in a minute. You want to go on a run together so you can beat me. Which probably won't be that hard unless we're doing sprints and I'm chasing a football. You want to eat a lot of food, which makes me love you already, and you're wearing an ugly pink dress for your sister's wedding when most people would tell her to stuff it."

Fat, you mean, I thought with a stab of fear. *I'm just not skinny and perky and ditzy like other college girls.* But the easygoing look in his eyes had nothing to do with judgment.

"Is that a good thing?" I asked hesitantly.

"Duh. Your healthy habits are motivating me to get back on it before spring training. I chub up a bit every winter when I'm not going to two-a-days or playing games every weekend. That's definitely a good thing." He slapped his stomach, which I imagined to be hitting rock-hard abs because I couldn't see below his shoulders.

"Spring training?"

Bradley was a football player? How had this never come into conversation before?

"Yeah. I'm attending college on a football scholarship. My parents run a farm so we never had a lot of money. I played sports to put me through."

My eyes widened. "You never told me that."

"Wasn't important."

"How have we not discussed it?" I asked, feeling incredibly stupid. "We've been talking for over three months now."

He shrugged. "It's the off season. Football is my life the rest of the year. It's nice to have a break. Besides, can I be honest?"

"Of course."

"Some people get weird about football players. We're not even that big of a college. I mean, it's not like we're going to get on ESPN or anything. I love football, but it's mostly just a method to help me get my MBA. But, I don't know." He shook it off.

"People get weird because you play ball? This is America."

He laughed. "Yeah, but there's all kinds of stereotypes. What I've liked about talking to you is that I'm not just a jock football player that likes to party and doesn't have any motivation for life outside the game. I want to own my own business. I prefer staying in over going out, I hate busy restaurants so I do a lot of take out, and when I go on dates, I hate it when girls wear dresses so skimpy I don't know where to put my hands."

No problem here, I thought.

"With this—" He motioned between us. "I'm just a guy who has never read *Frankenstein* and feels pity for the girl who has to wear a really pink bridesmaid dress."

He gave me a pointed gaze full of pity, and I burst into laughter.

"But seriously," he continued, "tell me more about this wedding and your sister, because based on what I've heard through your messages, I can't *wait* to see how it all plays out."

Chapter 34—Buy a New Shirt

Bradley and I video chatted for three hours. In the course of those three hours, we completely forgot to talk about the book *Frankenstein.*

I sailed through the next week on a strange oblivion, humming in the middle of workouts, easily rejecting vending machines that used to whisper at me when I strolled past. I stayed within my calorie goal, and started writing three short stories.

All of which I deleted entirely before I finished a first draft.

"Lexie, you've already missed the deadline for two of the smaller competitions," Miss Bliss admonished with a *tsking* sound. Her massive horn-rimmed glasses reflected the glare of the fluorescent light of her office. "I can't help but feel suspicious that you don't *really* want this internship."

The heady feeling I'd been carrying around with me for the past week crashed into smithereens.

"I want it," I said. "I want this internship more than anything. But I can't find any inspiration to write. Some of the prompts are really terrible."

"I've read some of your work before; you're good. Good enough to win at least one. Even *that* would add something to your resume."

"But I wasn't under pressure when I wrote those other pieces. Besides, I've already submitted them to competitions in the past and they didn't win. I don't want to waste the entry."

"Well you're under pressure now. You're going to have to figure it out." She pinched her lipstick-smeared lips together and appraised me with the narrow eye of an owl in contemplation. "Writer's block doesn't just *happen,* you know. There's almost always a reason for it. You must not be looking in the right places or writing about the right things. What are you passionate about?"

Chocolate. Food. My thoughts flickered to my workout that morning, when I'd finally run three quarters of a mile without stopping on the treadmill. Writing a story about Bradley would be way too creepy.

I shrugged. "A lot of things?"

Miss Bliss leaned back in her old chair, which groaned beneath her shifting weight.

"Figure out what you *are* passionate about and the story will write itself."

Writing itself wasn't new to me; I'd often conjured up stories in my childhood and played them out on paper. When Dad and I weren't binge eating and watching the latest football game while Kenzie and Mom did crafts, I was reading. Devouring romance books and picturing myself as the simpering, beautiful, skinny female swept away by the dashing rogue. But those weren't real, and I'd never written to win anything.

"Yes, Miss Bliss," I said, grabbing my bag by the strap and rising. "I'll work on it."

She pulled her glasses down until they rested on the tip of her nose. "Do that. And you're looking good, by the way. Don't know what you're doing, but keep it up. Oh, and buy a new shirt. That one's drowning you."

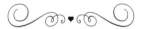

"Relax, Lex. It's just shopping. Nothing is going to bite you, you know."

Mira walked into the mall next to me wearing a bright red and pink muumuu with orchids on the front.

"Mira," I said, pulling open the main door and stepping into a white tiled world that smelled like caramel corn and french fries. Of course we *would* go in the food court on a Saturday, when delicious smells bloomed like early spring flowers. "You're looking really good."

Her gowny dress hid it, but her arms and shoulders had definitely slimmed down. She didn't waddle with a side-to-side, unbalanced gait anymore.

"Thanks. Going off Diet Pepsi helped—don't tell Bitsy—but that doesn't mean I still wouldn't kill for a pretzel."

We hurried past the pretzel stand and into the closest department store. The subtle reminder of giving up Diet Dr Pepper stung a bit, but not as badly as I thought. After the first week of headaches and withdrawals, I'd slowly been forgetting about it.

"Do we have to do this?" I asked with a twist of my stomach. I hadn't been shopping on purpose in . . . well . . . far too long. Mira cast an eye at my shirt, which, admittedly, hung a bit loose.

"You look like you wrapped yourself in your old drapes."

I was about to protest but she ignored me and headed for the plus size section. I skimmed the tops of the racks, but didn't see any familiar faces to hide from. I'd never shopped outside of the plus size section in my life, and felt shame every time I walked through.

"What pant size did you wear before?" Mira asked, perusing a display of shirts designed with bright tropical flowers. I quickly steered her away. She grabbed a few shirts along the way, draping them over her arm.

"Uh, size eighteen was the last pair of jeans I remember buying, but they . . . were a bit tight."

Mira continued her path, plucking blouses, pants, jeans, dresses, and skirts off every rack she passed. She dumped a bundle of clothes into my arms and shoved me into a dressing room.

"Try these."

"But—"

The door closed behind her with a firm *clang*. "Just do it, Lexie."

Obedient, but still grumbling under my breath, I slipped out of my pants and grabbed the first pair I saw. Out of habit, I avoided looking at the size, put my back to the mirror, and quickly pulled the jeans up, bracing myself for the usual tightness in the thigh and bulge of my stomach spilling over the too-small waist. Except the pants slid easily over my legs. And they buttoned.

I blinked several times. "Wait, what?" I whispered.

"Well?" Mira asked. "Let's see!"

My fist fit in between my stomach and the zipper, finding lots of room to spare. I checked the legs, which hung loose, and finally the butt, which sagged a bit in the back.

"Hold on," I called, and scrambled out of the pants. My hands shook when I finally found the tag. "Eighteen. It's a size eighteen."

"Did you take them off?" Mira asked, stalking up until her feet waited on the other side of the door. "I want to see!"

Shocked, I stepped back into the pants, pulled them up, and opened the door. Her outraged frown turned into a question when she cocked her head to one side and braced her hands on her hips.

"Well, *those* are certainly too big. We're going to have to go down a size. Try the sixteens."

Sixteen? I thought in disbelief as I shut the door. *I haven't worn a sixteen since . . . early high school.*

The nervous flutter in my gut turned to disbelief, and then raw emotion, when the size sixteen jeans easily slid up my legs. They felt snug, but not sickeningly tight, and left no bulge in the waist. I sat down, buried my face in my hands, and started to cry.

"Lexie?" Mira charged into the dressing room. "What's wrong? Is everything okay? Why are you crying?"

"Because they fit."

She put a hand on my shoulder. "That's no reason to cry! That's a happy thing, Lexie."

"They've never fit before. It feels . . . *I* feel . . . so good."

Mira sat on the bench next to me with a long sigh and the two of us stared at the white wall while I sniffled, trying to get my emotions under control.

"It does feel good, doesn't it?" she asked with a little smile.

"I never want to go back, Mira. I never want to feel the way I used to. I never want to hate myself again."

"That's the greatest part of all this, Lexie. We don't have to."

My legs looked remarkably thinner now that I didn't have miles of fabric around them.

"Yeah," I whispered, returning her teary smile. "I guess we don't."

Chapter 35—Death. Like Death.

"Whoa, Lexie. You look great. Did you get a new outfit or something?"

Megan walked up to me in the gym later that week with a wide grin, her hair swinging in a braid. I glanced down to my outfit with a sheepish smile.

"Mira made me go shopping." I gestured to Mira, who puffed away on the elliptical and waved. "We bought me some new workout clothes. Are they too tight?"

The new shirt felt like it hugged my shoulders and chest, but Megan shook her head.

"No way. It slenderizes you."

"Thanks."

"Hey, Dana had to bail on me today, so I just finished my workout early. I'm thinking about going for a run. Want to join?"

I reared back. "A run?"

"Yeah."

"You want *me* to run with *you?*"

"Of course."

I bit my bottom lip. "Well . . . uh, I don't really . . . my run is more of a . . ."

"I've seen you run." She motioned to a treadmill. "If you can run on the treadmill, you can definitely run outside. There's a little park in back with a loop that is exactly a mile."

My throat had gone dry, so I had to clear it before I could form a semi-coherent response. "I've never run a mile before."

"It's a beautiful day to start."

Her optimistic attitude would have been infectious if we were talking about drinking Starbucks vanilla bean Frappuccinos. But running?

Really?

"I could try," I said, clarifying with a quick, "but my run is more of a wog. Less gazelle and more hippo."

She shrugged. "I'm not running for time. Sometimes it's just nice to be outside exercising with someone."

Surely horns would grow out of her head any minute now.

"Enjoyment?" I scoffed, snorting. But her expression didn't change, so my amusement quickly crashed. "Oh," I whispered. "You're serious. You really do enjoy running."

"I do! Now c'mon. Let's just try it."

I hesitated, glancing to Mira, who had zoned into an episode of *The Golden Girls* while sweat poured down her face.

"Okay," I drawled. "But this could get ugly."

Megan led me to a small park behind the gym with a winding path that disappeared into naked, snow-covered trees. At least I wouldn't get massive pit stains from the heat.

Megan stood on one leg while stretching the other, pressing her foot into her butt while holding the ankle. I imagined myself trying, but would likely fall flat on my face.

"So what's the secret?" I asked, mimicking her actions as she stretched her arm across her body.

"The secret to what?"

"Enjoying running?"

She laughed. "Practice. You'll hate it at first, but just keep going. The more you do it, the easier it becomes. Pretty soon, it's kind of a Zen thing."

Megan definitely had a few more hippie tendencies than I, but she also had a lot more muscle and a smaller pant size, so I decided to believe her.

"I'll let you set the pace," she said, starting to walk. "The path loops around to make a mile."

I started slow. Running under my own power, and not with the guidance of the speed control on the treadmill, was so different that at first I felt disoriented. The bottom of my shoes scratched the cement as I shuffled along.

"This is a good pace to start," Megan said after a minute or two.

"A lot of people start too fast and wear out, but you should be able to maintain for a mile."

I said nothing. My heart was already beating hard against my ribs, and blood rushed through my arms and legs. Pretty soon, the gym disappeared and nothing but a winter landscape of brittle tree branches and piles of snow surrounded us.

"Wow," I said in between pants. "It's . . . so pretty . . . out here."

Megan touched a nearby twig as she passed, not even showing signs of heavy breathing or fatigue. The goofy smile on her face meant she really *was* enjoying our little jaunt. I drew in another lungful of air, trying not to gasp. Some mysteries in life would never make sense.

"Being outside is one of the best parts of running. It introduces you to things you may have never seen before."

The fresh air *was* nice. Perhaps my lair wasn't really the "safe place" I'd thought. Compared to this sunshine and the wintry beauty of the trees, the basement seemed more like a dungeon. Running wasn't the worst thing so early in the morning.

"How you feeling?" Megan asked a few minutes later.

"Fine," I said, panting. "Fine."

My lungs felt like they were on fire, so I dropped the speed down just a notch. Megan followed suit without a word. I had to blink several times, fighting a sudden watering in my eyes. My stomach hurt from breathing so hard.

"How much . . . longer?"

"Halfway."

My eyes bugged out of my head. "What? That's it? Aren't we . . . halfway to . . . China?"

She slapped me on the shoulder. "You got this, Lex. Just keep going. It's all in your head, really. Think of how good it's going to feel to finish a mile!"

The euphoria of running that she chased didn't exist in my world, so I pictured a hamburger hovering just in front of me. Onward I trudged—because what I was doing could hardly be called a run—feeling a sudden kinship with the pioneers of the Oregon Trail. Their life must have sucked.

"Quarter of a mile left. Look! You can see the back of the gym,"

Megan called, pointing through the tree branches ahead. The sidewalk had looped around again, leading us back. The beauty of nature didn't even appeal to me anymore. All I could focus on was the desire to slow down. But if I slowed at all, I'd stop completely.

I wouldn't do that because . . . well . . . I actually *did* want to see if I could do it. I'd never run a mile. Not even in gym class, where I'd pretend to sprain an ankle or just walk. I'd run three quarters of a mile on the treadmill but that had been easier because I'd been watching *Jeopardy* at the time.

"So close!" Megan called. I panted and snorted and puffed and huffed until I wondered if I'd pass out. A stitch drilled into my side just as I came up to the final stretch.

"Argh! My side."

"Breathe through it," Megan said. "Just take in extra-deep breaths."

I wanted to punch her and tell her to take her own deep breaths—I wouldn't have been this miserable if she hadn't popped up that morning—but that would have cost extra energy, so I settled on imagining a hamburger again. Perspiration dropped down my cheeks.

How did anyone enjoy this torture?

"Ten more steps! Ten more!"

Megan danced ahead of me. Once my feet crossed our starting point she threw her hands in the air and hopped from side to side.

"You did it! You ran a mile!"

I doubled over. A slight wheeze accompanied every breath. Megan slapped me on the shoulder again.

"You did it, Lexie! I knew you could."

My scalp tingled and heart pounded as I drew in breath after breath, grateful when the burning in my chest began to subside.

"Isn't it the greatest feeling?" she asked. "I love it!"

"Death. Like . . . like death."

She had the audacity to clap and giggle. The desire to punch her had started to fade, but only slightly.

"Why was that so much harder than the treadmill?" I asked, straightening once I had regained my breath. "I . . . that sucked."

"Because you have to pace yourself, and you don't have anything distracting you. Running is a mental game as much as a physical one."

I glanced back at the trail. "I did it though," I said, finding the first semblance of a smile. She grinned back.

"Yeah, you did."

I, Lexie Greene, had just run a mile for the first time in my life. I fell backwards into a snow bank, arms spread wide, and laughed.

♥

Chapter 36—The Most Wonderful Thing

♠

Bits of snow clung to my hair when I walked in the house the next week. My cheeks, pinched from the cold, prickled when a rush of heat blew across my face. Mom stood at the bottom of the stairs holding a handful of fake flowers in one hand and an empty vase in the other.

"Oh, hi Lexie. I didn't realize you were out. I thought you were in the basement."

"Bitsy challenged us to take more walks at our meeting yesterday," I said, unwinding the scarf and setting it on the coatrack. "Since Kenz and I didn't have Zumba tonight, I thought I'd stroll around the neighborhood."

Mom blinked a few times. "Really?"

"Yeah."

"That's . . . that's great. I've been meaning to tell you that you're looking really good."

I shrugged my coat off. "Oh, thanks."

"Are you feeling good too?"

"Yeah." If I admitted that being healthy felt better, would Mom rub it in my face? Would she say *I told you so?* "I actually . . . I don't think I've ever felt this good before."

She gave me a careful smile. "That's great."

Mom and I didn't speak much on a daily basis, outside the trivialities of who was going to go grocery shopping or do the chores. Kenzie had Mom wrapped up in wedding plans, and I avoided confrontation by hiding downstairs. It had been a while since the two of us had really been in the same room. Not to mention I had a history of being sensitive about anything regarding my weight, so I'd purposefully avoided talking to Mom about anything related to the *Health and Happiness Society.*

We stood in the awkward silence for an interminable minute.

"How are the wedding plans?" I asked.

"Fine." She shook the plastic flowers in her hand. "Just trying out a few possible arrangements. I'm not really sure how to organize flowers into a bouquet, but Kenzie's determined to save money on fake flowers."

"Do you want some help?"

Her eyebrows rose. "From you?"

"Sure."

"Uh . . . yes. I'd love some."

A plethora of fake flowers, crunchy green balls, a hot glue gun, and different vases littered the table in the dining room already. Most of the flowers were a light rosebud color, while others blazed hot pink. Springs of baby's breath and a few white roses sat on the counter as the only non-pink options.

"There's no rhyme or reason to it, really. I told Kenz that I'd put together a sample of bouquets, and she could pick which one she liked. Start putting something together, if you'd like."

I picked up a light pink tulip and paired it with baby's breath. Mom stood across from me on the other side of the table while we worked in silence.

"How are your classes going?"

Good, I thought of responding, the way I did whenever she asked in passing. But tonight I sensed a dropping of the walls and decided to be honest.

"Not bad, but I'm frustrated with my advisor, Miss Bliss."

Mom seemed to hold her breath. "Oh?"

"I'm applying for a competitive internship with Delta Publishing in New York City, and she wants me to submit to writing competitions. She thinks if I show I can write then I'll have a better chance of getting the job."

"New York? I had no idea you were looking at an internship."

A sheepish sense of shame crept over me. I hadn't exactly been open lately. "Yeah, just thinking about it."

I set down the flowers I'd compiled so far and stood, headed for the fridge as if on autopilot. There had been an old doughnut of Kenzie's earlier this morning that I had avoided but would taste wonderful now.

Chocolate frosting will make this conversation with Mom less awkward.

Light spilled into the kitchen when I pulled open the fridge. Just as I reached for the doughnut container, I stopped.

What am I doing?

Last time I'd had an encounter with Mom, this exact thing had happened. I turned to the ever-ready arms of food and binged almost uncontrollably. Mom kept working, oblivious to the pause in my universe, the shift in time, as my frozen arm remained halfway into the fridge. Did I want to go down that path again?

No. I grabbed a water bottle instead. *No. This time, I'll deal with my emotions. I won't eat them.*

"Want a water bottle, Mom?"

"Sure."

When I returned *sans* food, she glanced at the two water bottles in my hand. Mom had never been good at hiding her surprise.

"Thanks," she said, accepting it. I twisted the cap off, chugged half of it—I'd forgotten that I'd been thirsty from my walk—and then returned to my flowers.

"Anyway," I continued, as if I had never stopped my explanation. "Miss Bliss wants me to submit my writing, but I don't know what to write about. Some of the competitions have writing prompts, but none of them appeal to me. She says to find something I'm passionate about, but . . ."

I paused. *I've never been passionate about anything except food, and look where that got me?*

"What about your father?" Mom asked. "You were so close to him."

A twinge of longing, perhaps pain, had come into her voice, although she tried to cover it with a forced smile. I stared at her in surprise.

"Write about Dad?"

She shrugged. "Why not? He meant the world to you, Lex. You were always glued to his side."

I studied the hurt on her face. "Mom," I said quietly, surprised to hear the words moving from my brain to my lips, "did you ever feel bad because I was so close to Dad?"

Tears rose in her eyes. "What do you mean?" she asked with a little laugh, although she almost choked on it. "I was glad you were so close with him. Heaven knows he needed someone who understood him. I never did."

"What do you mean?"

"Your father was a good man, but he wasn't perfect. Instead of talking through our problems, he would just eat. And eat. A lot of things went unsaid because of it. Instead of spending time together, he wanted to be out to dinner or watching his favorite TV show. We didn't *do* much."

I'd always brushed Mom off as an emotional creature growing up, but suddenly I saw it in a different light. All those nights sitting in front of the TV with Dad, watching games on Saturday, spending half of the baseball games we'd attended trying out different food vendors.

Where was Mom during all this?

I opened my mouth to say something but shut it again. "I had no idea," I whispered, dumbstruck. "I just . . . I just thought that you didn't like Dad. That you weren't attracted to him because he was overweight."

"Not like him?" she asked. "Lexie, I loved your father no matter what he weighed. But food became his mistress. And me? I . . . I don't know what I was. Then . . ."

Her frightened gaze finished the rest of her statement. *Then he dragged you down that road with him.*

He did. Dad certainly had taught me how to cope with life— or not cope with life—through food. All that time Mom had been trying to put me on diets, telling me that I needed to lose weight, she'd really just been terrified that I'd end up like Dad: obsessed with food. Dad had been my hero. My best friend. The one who understood. The guy who didn't care what others thought. But now I realized that perhaps he was just as messed up as me all this time.

"I'm sorry," I said, meeting her watery gaze. "I had no idea, Mom."

A tremulous smile crossed her lips. She reached over and took my hand. "It's okay, Lexie. You didn't know. You were just a girl."

"I won't do what Dad did to you. Well . . . maybe I did in the past. Okay," I admitted reluctantly, my forehead furrowing, "I've done to you *just* what Dad did, but I won't anymore. Everything is different for me now. I'm getting healthy in lots of ways. I'm . . . going to be happy too. Happy with me, happy with my size, happy with my life. And . . . I'll try."

A tear dropped down her cheek as she squeezed my hand.

"That sounds like the most wonderful thing I've ever heard, Lexie girl. The most wonderful thing."

Chapter 37—Bradley is Here

"Hey, Lexie, can you bring out the éclairs?"

Pat called to me from the front bar of Lucky's, where the Friday night regulars had started filtering in to watch the latest sports highlights. I'd never minded working Friday night, as it gave me a solid excuse for not having a date. These days, however, I was beginning to wish I *did* have a date. One that went by the name of Bradley.

July seemed so far away, and yet, not far enough.

"Got it!" I called back, shutting the mega-fridge and purposefully keeping my eyes away from the tasty pastries that one of the regulars had brought by for their *Boys Night Club* tonight. Before, I would have stolen one before I brought them out—and no doubt they bought one for me because they were nice like that—but this time I didn't bother. I'd officially been losing weight for two months. My size sixteen jeans wore so comfortably now that just a few more Zumba classes with Kenzie and wogs with Megan would put me in a sleek fourteen. Besides, two more weeks would bring another weigh-in. I might not be focusing on the number *as* much, but I still wanted it to go down.

My phone buzzed as I walked past it on the back counter, but I ignored it, beckoned by the call of men screaming at the TV in the front. By the time I made my way out of the back, all seven of them were throwing balled up napkins and shooting straw wrappers at the TV while banging their fists on the bar.

"Here you go." I plopped the éclairs in the middle of the bar and grabbed my apron from the hook just below the counter. They applauded.

"Lexie?" called one of the old Irish men, a hint of a brogue on the edge of his voice. "Is that you?"

"What happened?" cried another. "Where are ya going?"

"She's lost weight."

"Yeah. She looks good. Leave her alone."

"Lexie, I'm free tonight!"

I laughed at their rising chorus and waved them off—secretly pleased that the old farts had even noticed—and turned my attention to the customers the hostess had just seated on the far side of the bar. Lucky's was filling up fast. I caught a glimpse of myself in the mirror and nearly cringed. I'd had to settle with putting my hair in a haphazard, loose bun on top of my head. Cooked cabbage stains smeared my apron, and I looked as tired as I felt.

"Well," I muttered, fishing for a pen in the pocket of my apron, "at least I'm not out to impress anyone."

A group of four college boys—no doubt football players by their large size—waited around a table in the back corner. I pulled my notepad out of my pocket as I approached. Usually I would have kept my eyes averted while I took their order—nothing was more awkward than being a chubby girl approaching a table of jocks—but tonight I didn't, and it felt good to even pretend like I had the same confidence Megan had.

"Welcome to Lucky's," I said with a smile. "What can I get you?"

"Whoa. Wait. Lexie?"

The man against the wall on the left straightened. My heart leapt into my throat. For one terrifying moment I was completely and utterly breathless.

"Bradley?" I whispered.

Those familiar pond-water hazel eyes crinkled with a grin. He shook his head in disbelief and nudged his friend in the arm. "Dude, this is the girl I was telling you about. The one I've been talking to that lives here? I can't believe it!" He turned back to me. "I had no idea you worked here. We were just looking for a place to eat tonight. I tried texting and calling but you never answered. I can see why now!"

He stood up, arms spread wide, and wrapped me a bear hug that would have entirely swallowed a lesser human. Football player was right. His shoulders were as wide as a barn in real life, and thick too. He had the look of being strong, like a corn-fed farmer boy that could move a water pipe but also eat half the table.

My pulse was thready and weak when I half-heartedly returned the hug, too stunned to do more than pat him on the back. I managed a smile, but it no doubt looked pained. Cabbage on my apron. I had cabbage on my apron and Bradley, the love of my life, was standing before my very eyes. Not only that, but he was everything I had imagined.

And more.

He pulled away, but kept a hand on my shoulder. It burned into my skin. "How late do you work tonight?" he asked. "We're in town for a friend for the weekend, but his thing is only tomorrow morning."

"Dude," one of his friends said. "We've got that game tomorrow night at—"

Bradley cut him off. "I could definitely hang out the rest of the time. What do you say? Let's do it."

"Really?"

He squeezed my shoulder. "Oh yeah. It'll be great. This is the best surprise yet."

But I'm not beautiful. I'm not skinny. How can you show any interest in me when I don't have makeup on and my hair is a mess?

"Lexie!" Pat called from behind the bar, glowering beneath heavy eyebrows. "Everything all right? You need anything?"

A defibrillator for my heart.

Pat glanced pointedly at Bradley, no doubt as shocked as I that some strange, rugged male would walk up and give me a hug. Bradley immediately dropped his hand and took a step back toward the table. I wanted to curse Pat.

"No, Pat. We're good here," I said, waving him off. He growled like a bulldog and continued wiping down the bar while the *Boys Night Club* howled at the TV, but kept his eyes on Bradley. I turned back to Bradley, needing nothing more than a minute to pull myself back together. "Let me take your orders and we'll work it out from there, okay? I . . . I'm in the middle of something in the back. I just need to, uh, finish it really quick."

Bradley grinned, effectively stopping my heart a second time. Those full lips.

"Perfect."

After hastily writing down what they wanted—I couldn't remember it even two minutes later—I handed the slip to Pat, asked him to cover for me for a minute, and disappeared into the back. I snatched my phone off the counter and ran into the bathroom, locking it behind me. Bradley had tried to call, three times in fact. Four text messages from him waited me, and I cursed myself for not paying more attention.

My fingers trembled as I sat down on the toilet and typed Rachelle's number. I ran a hand through my already wild hair.

"Pick up!" I hissed as it rang and rang. "Oh, please, Rachelle!"

"Hey. Aren't you working tonight?"

"Rachelle!" I screeched. "Oh, you're there. You have to help me. The worst possible thing in the world just happened."

"You binge ate a bunch of Krispy Kremes? Oh, no, that was me, sorry. I'm depressed about not having a date again and—"

"Rachelle, listen! Bradley is here."

Silence followed my declaration.

"What?"

"Bradley! The love of my life? The hottest man on the planet? Remember?"

Tears sprang to my eyes when I saw something out of the corner of my eye and pulled a straw wrapper from my hair. I'd been dreaming of this moment with Bradley for months, and now it went down on a random Friday night with cabbage and straw wrappers and a still-chubby Lexie who wouldn't measure up.

"Seriously?" she asked.

"Yes! He just gave me a hug and it was . . . it was, you know, *perfect*. He's beautiful and perfect and I'm not, and I can't stop shaking."

To my consternation, Rachelle started to laugh. And laugh. And laugh. "Oh, Lex," she cried, giggling. "That is too much!"

"What do I do?"

"What can you do?" she asked. "Just roll with it. Go talk to him. You're wonderful, Lexie."

"But I'm not skinny yet! I was supposed to be skinny and hot and—"

"And you've learned nothing so far, have you?" she asked, stopping my frantic tirade. "Lexie, I thought losing weight wasn't about that for you anymore."

"It . . . it wasn't. But that doesn't mean that—"

"It doesn't mean that you're worth any less just because you aren't fitting some kind of picture in your head, right? Look at you. You look fabulous. You're wearing a pants size I haven't worn since middle school. Not only that, but you're figuring your life out. And you're glowing. So what if Bradley shows up unexpectedly? At least now he can meet the real Lexie. If you're chasing a dream of how everything *should* go, then you're going to chase it forever. Because, news flash, it never goes the way it's supposed to. Deal with it."

My pounding heart calmed. "You're right," I whispered. "You're right."

I could picture her rolling her eyes. "Duh. I'm always wise after consuming half a dozen Krispy Kremes. Okay, fine. I ate nine. Look, Lex. You have an awesome opportunity here. Don't waste it because you think you know what Bradley wants in a girl. You don't know him. You know a dream of him that you've conjured up in your head. Maybe he's a douche bag in real life. Go meet him and figure out if *he* is good enough for *you*."

After saying thanks and promising to update her, I ended the call and stared at the frightened girl in the mirror.

"Okay," I whispered. "Let's do this. Let's face Bradley for real this time."

Chapter 38—Class and Taste and Experience

"**Hey, Lexie,** you need me to take care of those guys for you?"

Pat met me by the massive fridge before I went back into the restaurant. The traitorous thought that I could tell Pat they were jerks from school and slip out the back momentarily flittered through my mind, but I chased it away.

Not spend time with Bradley? Madness.

"No, no. One of them is an . . . unexpected friend, I guess you could say."

Pat studied me with a bulbous eye for a second before giving in. "I took their drinks over and they seemed okay, but you never know. Not sure if they're staying for food or what. The *Boys Night Club* is getting a bit rowdy, so I may have to send them off. You sure?"

"Yes." I smiled. We'd had a few incidents with drunk men getting frisky in the past, so Pat had become a protective kind of papa bear whenever the nights became busy. "Thanks though, Pat. They won't be a problem."

"Okay. But you just tell me if I need to knock some heads or something."

Just my own, I thought. *So I know I'm not dreaming this.*

When I made it back into the front, the *Boys Night Club* was screaming at the TV, eyes already becoming bleary. One of them waved an éclair around, scattering custard over the face of his friend. Although I wanted to hide behind the bar and pretend to do something else—anything but talk to Bradley in this awful state of hair—I headed to his table again.

Wonderful, I thought as I approached, catching another glimpse of myself in the mirror. *I still haven't straightened my hair or cleaned the cabbage off my apron.*

But when I walked up, Bradley was sitting alone, lounging against his chair. He straightened when he saw me.

"Hey, girl."

"Where did everyone go?" I asked.

He glanced at the empty table. "Oh, them. They uh . . . they scattered for a while. I'll meet up with them later. No big deal."

"Oh, right. Well . . . can I get you anything?"

He leaned forward. "I'm good, don't worry about me. When do you finish your shift?"

"Not for three more hours."

"Oh, that's it? Sweet. I'll wait."

My eyebrows shot up. "You'll wait? For me to get off work in three hours?"

"Yeah." He shrugged and motioned to the bar with a jerk of his head. "Go do your thing. Have you had dinner yet? We'll go get something when you're done. Is that okay?"

"Are you . . . are you sure?"

He smiled and my heart oozed into a pile in my shoes. "Lexie, I'm always up for food with a beautiful girl. Waiting three hours is not a big deal, I promise. Go work and let me know when you're done."

I returned the smile, my heart pounding so fast I felt light headed. "Okay. I'll . . . uh, just let me know if you need anything." I turned back around in disbelief. "Really? Are you sure?"

"Go!" he called, laughing. "I can handle it."

The next hour passed with the vague awareness of him watching me every now and then as I interacted with customers. Despite my ugly, dirty apron, I was glad to have something to wrap around my body and hide my imperfect torso, making me feel like I could hide behind something. Lucky's had filled up, so I hardly had a spare minute to keep his Dr Pepper filled let alone chat.

"All right, George," I said to one of the *Boys Night Club* members as I plucked a half-eaten éclair from his waving arm before he smacked me with it in the face. "Hand over the éclair and let's call you a cab. I think you've had enough tonight."

I put a hand on his back to guide him off the chair, but he didn't budge.

"Lexie," George slurred, his fingers still pinched as if he held the pastry. Pat glanced over, but I waved him off. He was dealing with the other drunk members of the *Boys Night Club*. "You're lookin' good."

"Do you want me to call your wife to come get you?"

He shook his head back and forth so many times I thought he'd throw up. "No wife. No wife. No wife."

"Let's go, then. There's a cab outside that can take you."

"No wife!" he yelled. "I'm alone, Lexie! I'm ALONE!"

"George, calm down, all right? Let's get you home. You'll feel a lot better."

"Alone," he wailed, grabbing my arm with a chocolaty hand. He stopped and set a bloodshot eye on me, appraising me with the glassy eyes of a man swimming in heavy liquor. "Hey, Lexie. Yer pretty cute. Why don't you come home with me?"

"No, thanks."

His hand tightened with surprising strength. I tried to pull away, but he gripped tighter. "Butwhynot? Imma man. Yer a woman—"

"George, let me go."

"Aw, c'mon Lex! I could show you a—"

"Hey George!" A large hand grabbed George's wrist and yanked his hand off my arm. The next thing I knew, a familiar set of burly shoulders stood between George and I. Bradley gently pushed me back out of George's reach. "I think you've had enough to drink, my friend. Let's get you outside."

Bradley grabbed George's shoulder and pulled him off the chair. He glanced at me over his shoulder with a questioning look.

"I'm fine," I said, rubbing my arm. "Thanks."

The attention of the other patrons faded as Bradley escorted George outside. I grabbed the four empty bottles littering the bar and walked back behind the bar, feeling a bit shaky, although it had nothing to do with George.

"Sorry, Lex," Pat said. "I was trying to get over there."

I smiled to reassure him. "No problem, Pat."

"Why don't you leave early?" he asked. "Things are slowing here. The *Boys Night Club* is all leaving. I can handle the rest."

"But—"

He shoved me gently to the back. "Go with your little, well, not-so-little friend. Seems like a good one."

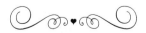

"Thanks for your help back there," I said to Bradley as we walked out of Lucky's Irish Pub together five minutes later. I'd replaced the dirty apron with a light jacket and managed to pull my hair into some semblance of order. My phone vibrated in my pocket every twenty seconds with a new message from Rachelle.

OMG what's happening?

You suck! Why haven't you updated me?

I'M DYINGGGGGGGG

Bradley waved it off. "Too easy, girl. So where do you want to eat?"

I motioned down the street. "There's a little diner down here that has really good chili cheese fries. Do you like chili cheese fries?"

He put a hand on the small of my back before we crossed the street. "A woman after my own heart. Let's do it."

Within minutes we were sitting across from each other in a booth, and I had a front row view of his beautiful hazel eyes. The waitress set two cups of ice water in front of us and left without another word.

"So?" I asked, already feeling the burden of a possible awkward silence. "What are you and your friends here for?"

"We have a few buddies that play basketball here. We were coming to hang out for the weekend and watch the finals. Pretty crazy that we walked into the pub where you work. I was hoping to see you but figured you were probably already booked this weekend, so I'm glad we could work something out."

You have no idea.

He leaned forward again. "Look, my buddy has a game tomorrow morning, and then there's another one in the evening, but I'm going to ditch that one because I think it's time you and I had an official date." He glanced around. "And not at a diner with chili cheese fries."

I laughed. "What? This isn't classy enough for you?"

"Class has nothing to do with it," he said with a grin that made my joints feel loose and slippery. "But taste and experience does. What do you say?"

So many thoughts ran through my head that I didn't even know where to start. I'd never been on a real date outside of the awkward high school blind dates Rachelle had forced me to endure so she could go out with all her random lover boys without inciting her mom's suspicion. I'd sit with my hands in my lap, my eyes glued to the TV, while she made out with whoever her tryst was at the time.

To say I was nervous, inexperienced, and terrified would understate it entirely. Not to mention that I had no idea what to wear.

"I say . . . yes."

He let out a long breath, and I realized I had paused in thought. "Whew. You had me worried for a second. I thought for sure you were probably already busy."

Too busy for you? Madness.

"By the way," he continued, "as a warning, I may or may not exploit this chance and take you to a horror movie with me just so I can appear macho and manly while you get scared. Think you could play along for the sake of my ego?"

"I'll simper and cry and throw myself into your arms."

"That would help a lot. I have to play this situation carefully, because I still want to be your date to your sister's wedding. No matter what happens between now and then, I've got to see this Pepto-Bismol bridesmaid dress."

"For blackmail purposes, I'm assuming?" I quipped, and he laughed.

"Definitely. Now the real question is this: how is writing going? Because we have to get you that awesome editing internship."

My stomach clenched. "Writing? It's . . . the same."

"Still nothing?"

To my surprise, I found myself telling him about talking with my mom, one-on-one, for the first time since Dad died. "Then she suggested that I write about Dad, just like you did. So . . . I don't know. I'm thinking about that now. There's just so much I could write. I don't know how to narrow it down."

His face had sobered. He took my life and concerns so seriously. Could I be interesting enough that he cared, or was he just being a nice guy?

"I think you need to write about what makes you happy, and talking about your dad always seemed to make you happy."

"Yeah. He was my best friend."

The waitress set a towering pile of chili cheese fries on the table between us. They had been Dad's favorite, so when I plucked one from the bottom and popped it in, I imagined being a little girl again.

"You're right," Bradley said after a few mouthfuls of fries. "This chili is amazing. But let's be honest. It's gotta go down with a disclaimer. I, in no way, take responsibility for how much I fart during our date tomorrow night? You good with that?"

I tilted my head back and laughed.

Chapter 39—Swanitude

My first official date with Bradley over chili cheese fries ended at two in the morning. By the time my alarm rang out at six, I was already awake, staring at my ceiling, in a near hyperventilation panic. Only one person that could give me any mental stability to face the day. I tossed off my covers, sent a quick text message, threw on my gym clothes, and grabbed my shoes on the way up the stairs.

Then I prayed Megan would show up.

As usual, the gym resembled a forgotten amusement park in the early Saturday morning hours. A few clownish people hung around, avoiding eye contact. I jumped on a bike and started pumping away as fast as I could, trying to out bike thoughts of disbelief, panic, and fresh blueberry waffles slathered in syrup.

"Are you okay, Lex?"

The voice of an angel appeared on the bike next to me twenty minutes later. By that time, sweat drenched my clothes and I gasped for air. Megan looked at me in concern, her eyes still sleepy, hair in the same braid, as always.

"You came!" I cried. "Megan, the worst possible thing happened last night and now I'm in a total panic. I need you to talk me down. Do whatever magic it is that you do when we talk and then I see the world differently. You ask me questions and then I have to think and suddenly the world is rose-colored instead of sepia. You know?"

Her forehead scrunched but if I left her confused, she didn't have a chance to say, because I launched into an instant replay of the night before.

"Cabbage stains," I repeated woefully, slapping my face with my hand once I'd finished the tale. "I had cabbage stains on my apron and a straw wrapper in my hair."

"Wow." She low whistled, her bike whirring. "That's pretty intense, Lexie."

"He's too perfect, right? He's way too perfect. Something has to be wrong with him. He has to be weird in some way. Right? I'm right."

Megan laughed. "Well, he did say he'd probably fart up a storm."

"Doesn't count," I mumbled, glowering at the bike display.

"Give it time, Lex. He's imperfect, of course. But that doesn't mean you have to find out all his flaws right away. Enjoy the honeymoon stage."

Now that the torrent of words had calmed, the cool grip of rationality crept in, and I felt sheepish. I cleared my throat. "Sorry I had you come here so early on a Saturday. I just . . . I just needed a friend."

A wave of guilt hit me for not calling Rachelle, but I had the innate sense to know Rachelle couldn't *really* help me the way I needed it, not in this. Megan waved it off.

"Don't worry about it. I love a friend that'll text me at six in the morning for an immediate, emergency, gym date." She smiled. "Besides, you need a girlfriend right now. Tell me what's really going on in your head. I have a feeling it has less to do with cabbage stains and more to do with something else."

My heart fluttered in a moment of hope. *This* was the Megan therapy that I needed.

"Well . . . it's just that I've had this planned in my head for months now, and I was wearing a black dress, with my hair done up, and I was the single most beautiful woman he'd ever seen. I wasn't at work or . . ."

"Wait. Who says you *aren't* the single most beautiful woman he's ever seen?" she asked.

I faltered over the automatic responses in my head. *Me. Common sense. I've never been beautiful. I'm not you.* Megan stared at me in expectation, and I realized she was waiting for a response.

"Me."

"Exactly. You're thinking for him. You can't do that in a relationship." Her eyes widened dramatically. "*Trust* me. If there's anyone on this planet that knows failed relationships, it's me."

"But Megan, I'm not you. I never have been. I'm not confident or . . . or put together or . . ."

"You're right. You're not me. You're Lexie," she said, interrupting a train of reasoning that would have surely led right into dreaming of bacon and pancakes. "And that is who Bradley met last night, and that is the girl he asked out on a date tonight. He didn't meet Megan and ask Megan out. He asked *you*."

The idea hadn't really crossed my mind that he might actually be interested in taking me out, and hadn't done so out of some weird sense of obligation. I swallowed.

"Yeah. I guess you're right."

Megan leaned back on her bike, her legs still spinning effortlessly beneath her. I hadn't even paid attention to anything but my jumbled thoughts while I rode, but I looked down to find that I'd just ridden over fifteen miles. A new record. Surprisingly, I felt better.

"Listen, Lex. You're losing weight and looking great. *Really* great. You're also dealing with crap in your life instead of eating your way through it. But your mind hasn't made quite as much progress. Worth isn't based off of numbers on a scale, and I don't think you've really realized that, even though you've made strides. Maybe this date with Bradley will help you see it."

"Definitely haven't let go yet," I agreed with a sigh.

Megan smiled. "Just remember to have swanitude."

"Yeah, right. I'm a swan."

Her eyebrows lowered over her eyes in indignation. "I'm serious, Lex. Tell yourself you're a swan. It's called Swanitude. Just keep repeating it all day. By the time you go out with him tonight, you're going to believe it."

I stared at her in disbelief. "Wait, you *are* serious."

She nodded. "It's how I got through my last breakup. Try it out. And don't get all crazy when you're prepping for your date, okay? Just go as Lexie. Don't pile on makeup and whatever. Just wear something you feel comfortable and beautiful in."

Just the thought of meeting Bradley that night for a date made butterflies flutter deep in my stomach. He'd been very gallant, very easygoing, and very sweet. Guys didn't just *do* that, right? *No,* I answered my own question. *Bradley didn't have to wait for me at work. He didn't have to send his friends away. That means something.*

That definitely means something.

I smiled over at Megan. "Thanks."

She laughed. "No problem. A little girl time sometimes straightens the world out. How about we end the morning with a few weight lifting exercises and then I'll take you out for a healthy breakfast smoothie to celebrate your date tonight?"

"This swan says yes."

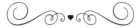

"Well," I said to my reflection later that night. "This is about to go down."

I followed Megan's advice and wore something comfortable, but still dressier than my sweats. My new pair of size sixteen jeans, a black t-shirt, and an unbuttoned gray cardigan jacket. Instead of going all out with my hair, I just washed it, fluffed it a bit, and wore it down. I hardly ever wore makeup, so I only put on mascara now.

At first I didn't recognize myself, and I stared at the mirror with a clenched stomach and mute disbelief. Who was this girl with cheekbones instead of a puffy face? My arms didn't stick out to the side like a Stay Puft Marshmallow doll. My torso had a more defined shape than just a bowling ball. I actually saw my eyes, instead of slits. It was the first time I'd really forced myself through a deep inspection of the accumulating changes since starting with the *Health and Happiness Society.*

"I'm a swan," I whispered. "A swan with swanitude[1]."

I smiled.

---

[1] Learn more about the #Swanitude movement at www.swanitude.com or follow on Twitter @swanitude

Chapter 40—Dirty Little Secrets

Bradley and I met for our date at Lucky's. While I was ready to throw my squishy, infatuated heart at him and tell him to keep it safe, I wasn't ready for him to accidentally meet my family.

"Hey," I said, walking up to where he sat at the bar, carrying on a bright conversation with Pat. The two of them were laughing over something. When Bradley turned to me, he grinned, his hazel eyes lighting up.

"Hey, girl. Ready to go? You look amazing."

"Oh, thanks. And yeah, I'm ready," I said, forcing nonchalance when I felt like I'd just been punched in the gut. His easy nicknames and blithe smile stole my breath. "Of course."

He held out a fist for Pat. They bumped fists in a manly departure. Pat sent me a thumbs up once Bradley's back had turned, and I smiled. Without Dad here, having Pat's approval meant just as much. Bradley's cell phone chimed as we walked out of the restaurant, then twice more in rapid succession. He ignored it.

"Is everything okay?" I asked, looking to his pocket. "Do you need to answer that?"

He waved it off. "It's just my friends."

Another chime.

"Sounds like they need you."

He pulled his phone out and silenced it. "They're just being idiots."

"Is this about the game you're missing tonight?" I asked. He stopped walking.

"Uh, yes. But . . . no. My friend Tyrone is playing in a basketball game tonight for March Madness, which is why I originally drove out. But this date is way more important."

I smiled, flattered despite myself. "That's really nice of you, but why don't we just go to the game?"

"Seriously?"

I shrugged. "Why not?"

"Because I'm taking you on a date."

"Fine, we won't stay the whole time. Just make an appearance, chest bump your buddies, and then we can go."

He looked at his watch. "I have reservations at Jim O'Leers at seven. It's six thirty now."

Jim O'Leers? I thought, my eyes widening. I'd never been to that restaurant, but if I remembered correctly, it cost at least thirty dollars a plate on the cheap end. A quick glance at our less-than-formal clothes confirmed that he'd either forgotten to tell me to dress up, or he hadn't done that much research.

We were off to an interesting start.

"So we'll stop by the game really fast," I said, brushing thoughts of fashion aside. "Jim O'Leers is by the campus."

He opened and closed his mouth, studying me with narrowed eyes. "I . . . that would be awesome. You sure?"

"Definitely."

"Wow. Well . . . great. You're awesome, Lex. There aren't many girls that would be so cool."

To my mortification, my cheeks flushed a bright red. "It's not a big deal, really."

"Not a big deal to you, maybe," he said, motioning to an old clunker car a few feet away with paint-chipped doors, which looked like they could fall off at any time. I thought it could be older than me. "Forgive my ugly steed. It's old and smells like football. Oh, come around to the driver's side. The passenger door doesn't open. Sorry. You good with climbing across? Okay, we'll make this stop at the game fast, I promise."

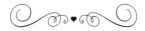

Forty-five minutes later, the annoyed glare of an extremely haughty butler stared both of us down. No doubt he resented the smell of popcorn and pretzels lingering from our visit to the basketball arena. My new jeans—while awesome and slenderizing—looked extremely out of place at Jim O'Leers amongst dressy cocktail gowns and polished shoes. Not to mention Bradley's flip-flops and cargo shorts.

"What do you mean you gave my reservation away?" Bradley asked, thumping his finger on the table. "I'm only a few minutes late, and I called ahead to—"

"Forgive me, sir, but restaurant policy states that if you have not arrived within ten minutes of your appointment, the table is given to another." He motioned to a queue of people waiting in line. "You are more than welcome to put your name on the wait list."

Bradley glanced over his shoulder and let out a frustrated breath.

"Let's just go," I said quietly. "Really. We'll find something else."

"Fine."

He put a hand on the small of my back to steer me back into the warm spring night. "Sorry, Lex. I should have left the game earlier. Tyrone was just on a roll, and I wanted to talk to him at the break."

"Oh, it's fine."

We approached his beat up car in silence. Bradley reached into his pocket for his keys and stopped. He patted his front pockets, then his back, and finally looked through the windshield with a groan.

"Damn!"

A shiny set of keys sparkled in the ignition. When I tugged on a door handle, it wouldn't budge. Bradley hurried around the other side of the car, but his had been locked. He slammed a fist onto the roof and pressed his forehead to the edge of the car.

"You've got to be kidding me."

While I felt bad for his pathetic state, I couldn't help the laugh that bubbled out of my chest, welling up with the realization that Bradley—Mr. Perfect himself—wasn't actually perfect at all. He looked up when I giggled. I giggled harder, and then leaned against the car and laughed. His eyes narrowed.

"I'm glad *you* can find amusement in this," he muttered, punching the car again, his eyes brewing into a stormy hazel. "I even left my wallet in there. Our first date and I've made it a bloody disaster."

I calmed my hilarity. "So let's walk."

"Walk?"

"Yeah. You use two feet. Put one in front of the other. We'll find some food."

"Where are we going to go?" he asked. "I don't exactly see you carrying a purse and my wallet is locked in the car."

"Well, no. I didn't think I'd need one. But that's all right. We'll find something." I looked at his car. "And a locksmith."

He lifted an eyebrow. "Seriously?"

Despite the fact that I didn't have any cash either, I grinned, elated with a sudden idea. "Don't worry. I got this."

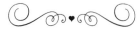

After calling a locksmith from my cell phone—and finding out it'd be at least two hours before he could meet us at the car—Bradley and I started walking. Twenty minutes later I stopped at a white gate.

"Here it is," I said, spreading my arms. "My new favorite place to eat."

He studied it with curious skepticism, having shaken off most of his bad mood while we walked. "It's a grass tiki hut."

I laughed. "Be adventurous. It has great food. My friend Megan introduced it to me. You should try their smoothies. C'mon. Cooper will let us eat and pay later."

To my relief, Cooper did remember me, and when I explained the situation, promised the food on the house. "Any friend of Megan . . ." he said, trailing off, and I wondered what kind of history they had that I didn't know about yet.

Bradley, looking a little like a defeated puppy, sat behind his strawberry and kale smoothie while island music tinkled in the background. "Listen, Lex," he said, leaning forward. "I'm sorry. I really wanted this to be a great date."

"It *is* a great date."

"No it's not." He rolled his eyes in a good-natured way. "We missed our reservation, I dragged you to part of a basketball game, my keys are locked in my car with my wallet, and now we have to bum food off of a hippie. This is not how I pictured it going. I won't blame you if you never answer my phone calls."

"Phone calls?" I asked, stirring my own smoothie.

"Yeah." He fiddled with the straw, pumping it up and down in the pink drink. "Once I leave. How else are we going to keep in touch? Facebook messages just aren't going to cut it anymore."

A little flame curled inside my chest, making me smile. "Oh, yeah, of course. I . . .I just . . . I didn't think you'd want to keep in touch."

My voice shrunk with the admittance. Somewhere deep in my head had been the idea that tonight was our only night. Cooper brought a plate of organic, non-GMO, Jamaican jerk nachos with locally raised shredded chicken in front of us. I smiled my thanks. He tilted his head, shot me an encouraging wink, and bowed away.

"Not keep in touch?" Bradley asked. "Are you kidding? Lexie, you're the most chill, easygoing girl I've ever met in my life. If this night had happened with Tami then—"

He broke off with the snap of his jaw shutting, pressing his lips into a firm line. My eyebrows rose. *Tami?*

"Secrets in the closet?" I asked, feeling a sudden empathy. I had my own skeletons rattling deep in hidden places, though mine tasted like chocolate bon bons.

"Man, I'm on a roll tonight," he said with a self-deprecatory sigh. "I can't do anything right. Should I just tell you all my dirty secrets since your friend is paying for our dinner, and you had to walk to a tiki hut just to get a meal?"

I smiled. "Ex-girlfriend?"

His face softened. "Yeah. She was a . . . a nightmare."

I leaned back. "Spill," I said, plucking a nacho off the plate. "I have all night long."

Chapter 41–One Big Monster

While I didn't have much—okay, any—dating experience, it seemed like a universal truth that one could learn a lot about a guy just by figuring out who he used to date. Bradley's nervous look as we shared a plate of nachos at the tiki hut already told me that learning about his ex-girlfriend Tami would be a very telling experience.

"It's simple," he said with a shrug. "We met in high school. We started dating as sophomores. At first it seemed great but it became ugly toward the end of our senior year. She didn't want me to take the football scholarship because she was worried I'd meet a cheer-leader and forget her. I deferred for a year, but it still didn't make her happy. I finally left for school despite her protests. Once I started college, she fell apart. She'd call me at three in the morning to see what I was doing, or yell at me for leaving her, or sometimes she'd randomly show up at football practice to make sure I hadn't lied. That kind of stuff."

My eyes grew with every sentence. I set down my sweating glass of water. "Really?"

He gave a lopsided smile. "Yeah."

"When did you break up?"

He exhaled a long breath. "Last October. I should have broken it off when I left for college, but I didn't. I felt too guilty and obligated. We had so much history together."

The calculation didn't take long. Bradley and I had met on Facebook in December. He hadn't been single all that long when we'd connected. And now he was finishing his junior year of college.

"Why didn't you break it off before October?" I asked. "Why stay with someone who obviously doesn't trust you?"

"Because I felt like I owed it to her. We'd been together for so long. She told me all the time that she deserved better, that I owed her more than leaving for college without her."

I grimaced. "Sounds abusive."

"Crazy," he corrected, trying to make light of it with a lopsided smile. Beneath the joking exterior, a true layer of uncertainty still lived. "She just needs someone that isn't me, and I wish her all the best."

His tone had a final edge that told me he'd say no more. Despite his forced nonchalance over the subject, I couldn't help but get the sense that he hadn't entirely moved on. Tami's influence obviously still lived on in his life. He leaned forward, recapturing my attention from the confusing cloud of thoughts.

"Listen, Lexie, I didn't bring Tami up to freak you out. I didn't really *mean* to bring her up in the first place. I just . . ." He hesitated. Our eyes locked and I found myself swimming in their muddy depths, feeling a bit lost myself. "I have a really good feeling about what you and I could be, but I don't want to screw anything up. I just need a little more time to figure out if I'm ready to make something happen. That is, of course, assuming you *want* anything to do with me."

My stomach caught. I stifled a little gasp of surprise before it surfaced. *I have a really good feeling about what you and I could be. . . assuming you want anything to do with me.*

Was he kidding? I wanted to grab his face and kiss him until he turned blue.

But you aren't ready either, something whispered from deep inside me. *Not yet. Not quite. No matter how much you want to be. There's still something left you haven't faced.*

The sudden, painful lump in my throat didn't swallow so easy.

"I see," I said when the silence stretched too long and I realized he was waiting for me to answer. He straightened, a flash of panic in his eyes, and held his hands up palms out.

"Look, I'm sorry if this was too straightforward. I just . . . Tami played stupid games with my head all the time so I promised myself that next time I felt interest in a girl, I'd be straight about it. And I think you're awesome, Lex. So here I am, being straight about it."

"I-it's not too straightforward," I said. "I don't mind."

His tense shoulders relaxed with a half-strength grin that looked mostly like relief. "I mean, we have just gone on the world's worst date, and you still haven't run away screaming. I figured that was a sign."

I grinned. "A good sign."

"So what do you say, Lex? Are you willing to give me a little more time to figure my crap out before we try to make something awesome? I won't ask you to bring more to the table than I can."

My heart hammered inside my chest. He didn't know the skeletons in my closet; he'd been too much of a gentleman to even ask. He didn't know that I was still a fat girl crying for her dad. Or that I still battled daily cravings for Little Debbie Cosmic Brownies and had to walk past Papa John's with my breath held so I didn't run inside and stuff my face with breadsticks.

Despite all my work with dieting and improving my health, there was still one growling monster in my closet that I had yet to confront.

One very big monster.

"I think that's a very reasonable request. Let's both work on our lives. I'm not . . . I'm not entirely ready either."

My response deflated his nervousness like a released balloon. The relief in his smile was so genuine that I couldn't help but smile myself.

"Thanks, Lex. I can't tell you how much better I feel."

Despite the small obstacle of admitting my history—my food-wrapper-riddled past—I felt the same way. Better. I couldn't let him truly know me without explaining that sugar and chocolate constituted a large part of my past. But I had the feeling he wouldn't care about it as much as I did.

You're not ready.

"Yeah," I smiled. "I feel better too."

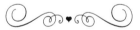

I returned from my date with Bradley with a thousand thoughts flying through my head.

Mom and Kenz were in bed, and the house lay quiet and dark. Instead of waking Mom up—although I knew she wanted to hear about Bradley—I left her a note. Normally I wouldn't have even bothered telling her, but the ice had cracked between us, and I wanted it to keep thawing, so I suggested we talk about it over breakfast.

I didn't bother turning on the light when I slipped into the basement lair. The wheels of my computer chair squeaked when I sat down. My monitor flickered to life, displaying my favorite picture of

Dad and me at a baseball game. I wore a backwards hat and my last true smile. Dad had died not long after.

One last monster, my inner voice reminded me. *You're not ready yet.*

No, I responded. *I'm not.*

Just behind the computer, tacked to my corkboard, was the flyer Rachelle had given me months before for the editing internship. The voice of my advisor, Miss Bliss, rang through my head.

What are you passionate about? Figure out what you are passionate about and the story will write itself.

My true passions were easily enough identified. Facing them all together, however, was not. I cracked my knuckles, opened up a word processing document, and put my fingers on the keyboard. Tonight, I would write. Tonight, I would face my monster.

Tonight, I'd start figuring out just who Lexie Greene really was.

Chapter 42—Abandoned

"**Lexie? Lex?** Seriously, wake up already!"

Someone grabbed my shoulder and shook me awake, pulling me from the deep reveries of sleep that held me captive. Images of Bradley whirled through my head, only to be replaced by Rachelle's quirked eyebrow and narrowed eyes.

"Why are you still asleep?" she asked. "It's almost two in the afternoon. You didn't even go to the gym this morning. Are you dying?"

I slowly straightened, surprised to find myself hunched over my desk, my back aching. I wiped my face with the back of my hand and struggled to clear my blurry vision. The imprint of a keyboard filled my face, and an endless stream of the letter *F* ran across the screen.

"I don't think I'm dying," I mumbled. "Though it probably feels this disorienting."

"When you didn't call me after your date with Bradley I got nervous. Mira texted me to ask where you were, said you hadn't been answering your phone. Your mom is at work, so I came to check on you. You're okay, right? He didn't slip you a Roofie or anything, did he? I'll kill him. I'll cut off his—"

"No!" I cried, batting her off. "He was a perfect gentlemen. It's nothing like that."

She plopped onto a nearby chair, her eyebrows raised in question. "So?" she drawled. "Why the heck are you still asleep?"

I pushed away from the desk. "I had inspiration for those writing competitions, so I started working on them last night." I squinted at the clock, as if that would help my brain figure out the numbers better. "I think I fell asleep around six this morning, but I can't really remember. It's all pretty blurry."

"Yeah, yeah. But was the date that good? Are you writing a romance?" She followed me to the bathroom, nagging me with questions the whole way. "Did he kiss you? Was it really romantic? Tell me everything! I have to live vicariously through you, remember?"

I slammed the door in her face before she could follow me in. "No. To both."

"Aw. Really? He didn't kiss you? He couldn't even make it romantic?"

Despite the less-than-exciting nature of my and Bradley's date, I found myself smiling over it. In its own way, it had been perfect. "He tried," I clarified, calling through the door. "The execution failed."

"So? Are you going to see him again?"

Her voice was slightly muffled through the door, but I could still hear the hope lingering in it. "Yeah," I said. "We will. But not for a while."

"What do you mean?"

"I mean that neither of us are ready yet."

She was standing right outside the bathroom door when I pulled it open, staring at me in open-mouthed astonishment. She waited so close to the doorway that our noses almost met.

"What? This is Bradley. Man of your dreams. The guy you've drooled over since December. How are you not ready for this?" Even though I stepped forward to move past her, she didn't budge. She shook her head. "Nope. You gotta explain. I'm *dying* here."

I sighed. "Fine. He's getting out of a complicated relationship, and I'm still figuring my life out, but both of us are interested. He sent me an email last night that said he was still planning on coming to McKenzie's wedding as my date, and we'll figure things out from there."

Rachelle's mouth dropped open. "That means you still have time to lose weight and get uber skinny! Lexie, this is awesome! You're going to get a Cinderella story."

The thought of having more time to lose weight hadn't actually occurred to me, and I didn't know to respond. A Cinderella story? What did that even mean?

"Yeah. I guess."

She stumbled backwards when I slid past, headed for my closet, where I rifled through my clothes to find something to exercise in. For the first time in my life, I had a head full of complicated thoughts that needed ironing out, and didn't think of food first. I looked forward to the Zen state that walking gave me where I could sort through the tangled web of decisions and ideas in my brain.

"What do you mean *you guess*?" Rachelle asked. "Lexie, you're going to keep losing weight. Then you'll wear a size eight and he'll have no choice but to love you."

"It's not . . . it's not like that anymore."

Rachelle plopped onto my bed, sprawling her arms wide. "You don't want to be skinny?"

"No, I just . . . I don't really feel like I *have* to be skinny for Bradley."

She scoffed. "You're so lucky. Finding a guy that doesn't care about your size. Do you know how hard that is?"

I stopped rooting through the bowels of my closet and turned to look at her. "It has nothing to do with Bradley. *I* feel like I don't need to be skinny for Bradley. But—" I hesitated, wondering how honest I should be, and decided to plunge in full strength. "But I do feel like I need to be whole."

She propped up on her elbows, appearing bored. "Whole?"

"Yeah. I'm so messed up right now. I just need to figure it out."

"Figure what out?"

"My brain. My heart. My life." I threw my hands up. "I don't know. Whatever *it* is. Then I'll give Bradley another shot."

"Is that what you're writing about? Your brain?"

"No. My dad."

Her eyes widened. "You're actually going to write about your dad?"

My heart felt fluttery and nervous. It had been one thing to spend seven hours pounding on a keyboard, writing everything out that I could remember about him. To acknowledge that open part of my soul to another person was another matter entirely. I wasn't ready to talk about it yet.

"Yeah. I finished what I wanted to do last night, so I'm going to take it to Miss Bliss tomorrow and see what she thinks of it. But in the meantime, I'm going for a walk. Do you want to join me?"

She stared at me, her eyebrows pulled low, her face puckered into deep furrows.

"What's happened to you?" she asked. I dropped my hands to my side and met her searching, if not frightened, gaze. "I feel like we're so different now. Like . . . like you're so far above me, and I don't know how to measure up. We've always been in this lifestyle together. I feel so . . . abandoned."

The bed creaked as I sat down beside her—I guess some things didn't change with weight loss—and I let out a sigh that blew my hair out of my face.

"I haven't left you, Rachelle. I'm just tired of wallowing and drowning."

She blinked rapidly, so rapidly that it almost hid the little sparkle of tears that had risen to her eyes. In all of our years as friends, I had never seen Rachelle cry. Not even when her dad packed up and left, or her mom had a heart attack at forty-three. Never.

"Yeah," she said, clearing her throat. "I guess I can understand that."

"Forcing the ghosts out of my closet doesn't mean we won't be friends anymore. It just means I won't feel so suffocated."

Rachelle smiled, but it was distant and weak. "I'm proud of you, Lexie. You're much braver than I am. There's so much wrong with me that I don't even want to face it, the way you are. Maybe one day I'll be like you. Anyway, let's talk about something else. What did you say about a walk? I guess I could use some sunshine and activity. Certainly isn't going to kill me, right?"

♥
....
Chapter 43—Not Great
....
♠

"**Well, Lexie.** I read over the file you sent me last week. The one with all the memories of you and your father."

Miss Bliss pulled her massive horn-rimmed glasses off to look me right in the eye, the way she usually did. Bangles of jewelry dripped from her neck in a gaudy display of turquoise and bright blue. Her gray bouffant had lost some of its puff, leaving her head looking smaller than usual.

"And?" I asked, swallowing back a lump of nervousness. Writing about Dad had exhausted me for over two days. Although a week had passed since the fateful all-night-binge-write, it seemed like an eternity. Getting her email in response to set up this meeting had been both terrifying and a relief.

"And I think it's your best writing, compared to the other short stories you showed me before."

I exhaled in relief. "Wonderful. I thought we could submit it to competition originating from the college here. It would look really nice on my resume to win something so close to home, I think."

She leaned back in her seat and bit her glasses with the front of her teeth, speaking through them with impressive clarity. "Listen. It's good writing, Lexie. But it's not great. Not great enough to win and help you get that internship, anyway."

Any sense of hope floundered, making me feel like someone had just pulled a string through my heart. I'd worked so hard on those memories. I'd dredged through every memory of Dad that I ever had, recalling some things I'd forgotten because they were simply too painful. At the time it had felt like putting my heart into a blender and turning it on high. Now Miss Bliss had just taken the lid off and pieces of me were flying everywhere.

"What? I-I don't understand."

"It's endearing, really, especially considering you lost him so tragically not long ago, but it is, in effect, just a stream-of-consciousness.

There's no real story. Sure, there's talent in the words and the phrasing, but no voice."

"The whole thing is in my voice!"

Miss Bliss didn't even flinch at the high-pitched defensiveness of my response. Her bright pink gum smacked between her teeth.

"No, it's not. It's a story being told. It's not *Lexie*."

I swallowed. "I don't know how to make it more Lexie. I . . . Miss Bliss this was the hardest thing I've ever written." My voice became small, even desperate. "It took everything I had."

We locked eyes. Miss Bliss's eyes softened infinitesimally around the edges.

"These are memories of a little girl that adored her father," she said, shucking aside the hard-nosed teacher. "You're not a little girl anymore, Lexie. You're a woman. A beautiful one. A strong one. One who has clearly endured a lot of trauma that you're just now realizing. You want to win this competition? Show me *that* girl. She's a hell of a lot more interesting than a few memories."

"But—"

"Real writing is raw and edgy. It's full of voice and honesty, and when you're doing it, it should hurt like hell. This is full of honesty and sure, some pain. But there's no grittiness, no voice. Give me a reason to read."

My heart pitter-pattered in my chest, and it took all my strength to keep from crying. How could it not be good enough? I averted my eyes.

"I don't know what else to write. I don't . . . I don't know."

Miss Bliss tossed a pile of papers at me. The title paper read *Dad and Me: Memories of My Father*. She'd printed off the manuscript I'd sent and edited it by hand. Comments, corrections, and the blood of the most ruthless college professor I'd ever met decorated the first page.

"Write *your* story," she said. "Not your dad's. I want to know about Lexie." She pointed at me with a pudgy finger. "This Lexie. The one sitting in front of me today."

A tingling rushed down my skin. I'd thought that the biggest monster inside me had been Dad and all the suppressed grief I'd pushed away with frosting and cake pops for the past couple of years.

The hope had been that releasing these memories would get rid of the toxicness inside me, but staring in Miss Bliss's determined eyes made me realize that I hadn't been exactly right.

I took the papers, mumbled a vague phrase of gratitude, and hurried out of her office before I erupted in tears. I didn't *want* to tell her—or anyone—about me. What was there to say? Talking about Dad had been hard enough. But myself? Who wanted to know about boring Lexie Greene?

Why did the monster have to be me?

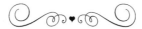

I lay in bed later that night, my body sore from a mile run with Megan, hugging a goose down pillow. While running the mile had become easier, it hadn't been any less torturous. No matter how often I did it now, I knew I'd never love running.

Miss Bliss's voice ran in a loop through my head.

It's good, but not great.

"You're not great, Miss Bliss," I growled in passive aggressive retribution. My phone rang, but I ignored it. When it rang a second time, I grabbed it.

"Yeah?"

"So . . . you didn't answer my phone call earlier today, and I thought there was a vague chance you might have walked into a volcano, so I thought I'd call to check on you again. Do I need to come rescue you? Does that pass as a totally non-weird excuse or am I pushing it?"

Bradley's joking nonchalance cut through my frustration. I relaxed my tense grip on the phone.

"Definitely a normal excuse," I said, flopping onto my back with a grin. "There are a lot of volcanoes around here."

"I know. That's why I was concerned. So what's up with you?"

"Uh, nothing, really."

"Doesn't sound like nothing. Didn't you have a meeting with your advisor today? What happened?"

My mouth bobbed up and down in hesitation, but deciding that talking it out would feel better, I explained my meeting with Miss Bliss.

"Ouch," he said with a little hiss. "She's tough."

"No kidding."

"But sounds like she also knows what she's talking about." I scowled, prepared to call him a traitor for siding with her, but he continued. "Look, Lex, you probably have a great story. One that I, quite frankly, would love to hear. What better way than to write it and win the internship?"

"No you wouldn't," I said immediately. "There's . . . there's so much you don't know about me."

He laughed. "Exactly. And I *want* to know more. So why don't you write the story?"

"Because I'm not exciting. I'm not like Megan. I'm not . . ." *I'm not skinny or adventurous or even daring. I'm just a girl addicted to food that hates running and dreams about apple fritters at night.*

"Wait, who is Megan?"

I sighed. "No one. Just a friend."

"Look, Lex, you don't think you're great, but maybe you just don't see it yet. Writing your story out would bring it together for you, I think. Maybe you'll start to see what everyone else sees, you know? Besides, what is it going to hurt to try? No one has to read it. If you hate it, throw it away and start something different."

He made it sound easy enough that my wall of hesitation started to crumble. I ran a hand through my hair.

"I could try, but it's not going to be pretty."

"Reality never is."

My heart hammered. "Are you sure you want to know everything about me? My past is not pretty either. I'm not perfect. I'm so far from it that it should frighten you."

I'm all jelly doughnuts, pecan logs, and cookie dough.

"Good, we'll be on even ground."

His disregard for the seriousness of this situation began to get on my nerves. Didn't he get it? He'd see how imperfect I was and run away. He'd learn that I used to binge eat hostess doughnuts, and I'd lose him. But wouldn't it be better that he ran away sooner rather than later? Spare me a little heartache so I could move on, forget he existed, and forge a new life?

"Okay," I said, blowing out a breath. "I'll write my story."

He applauded, then swore under his breath as I heard something clatter in the background. "Sorry, just dropped my dinner. That's awesome Lex. I'm really proud of you. And, more important, really excited to read what you come up with. Now, let's talk about how March Madness ended. I believe we had a bet, and you lost."

Chapter 44—Good Enough

The day after talking to Bradley about writing my story, I felt the deep pangs of a hunger stirring that had nothing to do with food, even though I dreamed of cinnamon rolls that night.

I woke up at 5:00 am to a growling stomach and a tempestuous head. I grabbed a banana and a piece of wheat bread on the way out and headed to the gym without Mira. Exercise cleared my head. I'd come far enough to know that eating my way through a problem only made me more fuzzy-brained, and pushed the problems off to deal with later. These problems couldn't be pushed away any longer.

Fifteen minutes later, with earbuds in and a spinning bike moving beneath my legs, I let my thoughts fly.

Write your story.

You're not a little girl anymore, Lexie. You're a woman. A beautiful one. A strong one . . . You want to win this competition? Show me that girl.

That girl lived amongst bon bons and starburst packages. She didn't like running. She refused to wear yoga pants because they'd show her lumpy legs. She wasn't perfect, and she held deep insecurities over all her many flaws. Why would Miss Bliss want to read about that Lexie Greene?

"Excuse me, can I ask you a question?"

A pair of blue eyes peered at me in question. A girl—who had to be a freshman based on her young, round face and naive eyes—sat on the bike next to mine. She wore a baggy, oversized shirt and a pair of sweats that probably once belonged to an older brother. They didn't entirely hide her large figure. Her blonde hair sat in a bun high on her head, showing the blush coating her cheeks.

I pulled my earbuds out. "Yeah, sure."

"I . . . I'm new here. Sorry to bother you, but I'd rather ask you than that guy at the front desk. Seems so humiliating that I don't already know how to work a bike. Could you . . . could you show me how to use this? I can barely push the pedals."

"Oh, yeah. The tension is probably high. Just twist that knob."

She turned the knob, and her legs started to flow freely. "Thanks," she said, exhaling with a relieved smile. "Even though there are not that many people here, it would have been embarrassing to just walk away."

I returned her smile. "Don't worry, I understand." The temptation to go back to my thoughts—which hadn't been all that revealing despite the exercise—came over me, but I ignored it. "So, you're new here?"

"Yeah!" she said, finding the easiest level she could on the bike. Her legs pumped with wild abandon. "My name is Anna. I don't really know that much about exercise, but I decided to try working out because I've put on a little more than the freshman fifteen. It's kind of embarrassing to work out at my size, so I came to the gym early before anyone gets here."

A wave of nostalgia rippled through me, and suddenly I didn't see Anna anymore. I saw a 259 pound girl wandering into the gym for the first time with no idea what it all meant. The baggy shirt, the hopeful desperation, the huffing and puffing with the slightest strain.

Had I really been just like Anna? So unaware? So naive?

I turned away before she caught me gawking. "What made you want to work out?" I asked, increasing the tension a little, needing something to push against.

"Oh, it sounds so dumb but . . . I actually met this guy. He doesn't even know I exist. I'm taking an art class with him, and he's just so cute. If I were to have any chance in the world then I need to look a little more appealing, I think."

Her voice faded into the background of my thoughts.

That's right where I started, I thought to myself. *I used to be just like Anna, back when I thought this was all about Bradley.*

Without meaning to, I caught a glimpse of myself in the mirror. My body was far from the svelte models that stared at me from the magazines at the side table. I still had padding everywhere, and still weighed over two hundred pounds, but the black workout capris I wore covered legs that had more muscle than flab. My abs didn't roll like a slinky anymore. And my face finally showed bone structure. The old Lexie Greene was slowly fading.

I'm not that girl anymore. I'm new. I'm better. I'm stronger.

For the first time in my life, I looked in a mirror and liked what I saw. A flawed girl who had a love affair with Great Harvest bread. A girl trying to get healthy. A girl that wanted to be in control of her life. I *liked* this Lexie. I stared at myself, twirling on the bike, face flushed, calves flexed, as if I had finally found a true reflection of me.

I'm Lexie Greene, I thought. *And I'm imperfect. I love food too much. I don't like to run and never will. And I am a swan.*

I am good enough.

". . . and then I accidentally spilled paint all over him. So he knows I exist, but it wasn't exactly an ideal way to introduce myself. Anyway, I think he prefers brunettes, but maybe I can change his mind if I could just lose some weight."

I pulled out of my thoughts. "You won't," I said, stopping the eternal spin of my legs. A feeling of empowerment and calm moved through me.

I am good enough.

"You don't think so?"

I looked at her with a wide smile. "You won't change his mind, and I don't know this guy at all, but he's not worth it."

Anna's mouth dropped open. "Wh—"

"Working out for a guy isn't worth it." I slung my towel over my shoulder, ready to take on the world. "You should work out for you, because you're worth it. Because you want to be healthy. Guys will come and go. Who cares about them?"

Anna floundered for a moment. "But . . . but I'm not pretty. I'm not confident. I'm not like you."

Her comment nearly stopped my breath. Isn't that what I'd said to Megan before? Was it possible that Anna saw the same lithe, easy confidence in me that I'd always admired in Megan? Is that what this feeling was?

"Yes, you are pretty and confident," I said, pulling my water bottle from the holder. "You just don't realize it yet. I come every morning at six with my friend Mira. If you come Monday morning at that time, I'll show you around so you don't feel so lost. I know how that feels. I'd show you today but I have something I need to do."

Her mouth dropped open. "Really? B-but you don't even know me."

"Yes I do. Better than you'll ever know."

I slung my gym bag on the bed and fell into my computer chair after sending a hasty text to Mira explaining I wouldn't make it to the gym with her. Sweaty, sticky, and feeling more alive than I ever had in my life, I closed all the Facebook browsers and opened a brand new word processing document. I grabbed a picture of Dad from where it hid in a drawer, taped it to my computer monitor and pulled in a deep breath. My fingers hovered over the keys for two seconds before I smiled and started to write.

Like any great story, it all began with Facebook.

Chapter 45–I Did It

I wrote for two weeks straight.

Spring break passed me by with all the force of a tornado, ushering May in like a hurricane. Except for Zumba with Kenzie, gym in the morning, and an occasional smoothie with Megan, I lived in the basement, writing, rewriting, and editing my contest submission. It was two in the morning, exactly fourteen days after meeting young Anna in the gym, that I sent Miss Bliss the paper.

Then I sat back, stared at the screen, and heaved a huge breath of relief. The contest submission date was three days away. I had to submit my application for the editing internship by June 15th, which meant I would just have time to hear back from the contest if I won and include it on my resume.

I *knew* the story was good. I could feel it deep in my bones. Not only was it honest and raw, but it hurt like hell to write.

Miss Bliss called me on my cell phone two days later. I didn't even know she had my number.

"In my office. Right now."

She hung up before I could respond. I veered away from my English literature class and cut across the grass for her office, pulling my almost-too-big jeans up before they fell around my ankles.

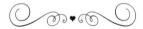

"Where have *you* been hiding?"

Miss Bliss tossed a marked up pile of papers on the desk in front of me. I caught them before they slid off and looked up.

"What?"

She motioned to the stack with a nod of her head. "That. Where has that been all this time?"

I held my breath. "You liked it?"

"No." She pulled her glasses off. "I loved it."

A little thrill ran through me. It didn't seem possible that Miss Bliss would approve of anything that I'd written. While I hadn't written to find her approval, it felt nice to have it all the same. "Really?"

"It's gritty and real. You didn't hold back, did you?"

"No."

"It shows. Was it difficult to write?"

The long nights of confronting my deepest insecurities rushed back to me like cannon fire. Difficult? It had been hell. Not only did I have to face my own issues, but I faced them knowing that other people would read it, judge it, critique it.

Knowing that when all was said and done, Bradley would know all my ugly secrets.

"Writing that was the hardest thing I've ever done, next to losing my dad."

"Good. That's how it should be. I stayed up all night reading it, so a fruit basket of appreciation would be nice. Fix up the punctuation errors and other things that I noted and get it submitted. Keep me updated. That is a winner."

I gripped the papers with both hands, feeling euphoric and breathless. No food on earth had ever made me feel this way before.

"Thank you, Miss Bliss."

She gave me a smile as slow as molasses. "Get out of here and edit your paper. It has to be turned in by midnight tonight. Oh, and Lexie?" She stopped me halfway out the door. I spun around, my eyebrows lifted.

"Yes?"

"What are you going to do for the title?"

I glanced down to the papers. I'd given the title a lot of thought, but couldn't decide. "I'm not sure. It's . . . it's not quite done, to be honest."

She tilted her head to the side. "Really?"

"I'm going to submit it like this," I said. "But the story isn't finished. Not yet. That'll happen in a couple of months."

She smiled. "Well, I can't wait to read the rest."

I did it.

My computer screen illuminated my face late that night as I sent a message to Bradley in the Facebook chat window. I had the windows open to let the cool spring air flood inside. If it hadn't been so close to midnight, I would have gone on a walk to enjoy the smell of juniper.

Bradley's response came fast. *Did what?*

Submitted my story.

The indicator of him typing paused for about ten seconds and then started again. *Really?*

Really. Miss Bliss loved it.

And how do you feel?

I hesitated this time. How *did* I feel?

Like a girl that finally knows who she is, I responded. My cell phone rang, and I picked it up without looking at who was calling so late.

"So who are you then?" Bradley asked. "Who is Lexie Greene?"

I pulled in a deep breath. "Well, uh . . . Lexie Greene is a girl that isn't perfect, that likes to eat, that has a repairing relationship with her family, and that prefers walking over running."

"Awesome. Do I get to read the story?"

"Yes, but, I'm going to ask you to wait."

"For what?"

I climbed onto my bed and lay on my back, staring up at the glow-in-the-dark stars that formed a whirling design.

"For the wedding. I want to be there when you read it, and it's not *quite* done, to be honest. I'm going to finish it after Kenzie's wedding."

"Okay."

His easy response, so unbothered by the request, relaxed me. "Really?"

"Yeah."

"Oh, well . . . that was easier than I thought."

"Shoot, girl. I'm just here to support you as a friend. I don't care when things happen, so long as they happen. Speaking of the wedding, it's coming up in two months. Have you gotten your bridesmaid dress yet?"

My nose wrinkled. "Ugh. No. Don't remind me."

He laughed. "I can't wait to see it."

"That is one thing that you will definitely have to wait for. I will not take any pictures unless I absolutely have to. It's hideous. Truly hideous." A yawn interrupted the rest of my response, and by the time I'd finished, I'd forgotten what I meant to say. "Anyway, I'm going to go to bed. Talk to you later?"

"Definitely. Sweet dreams, Lexie girl."

I'd no sooner shut off my phone and emitted a dreamy sigh when the basement door opened, spilling a sliver of light down the stairs.

"Lex?" Kenzie called down. "Hey, you there?"

"Yeah. What's up?" I called back.

"Are you busy tomorrow?"

"Not especially."

"Great. Your dress came in. They need you to try it on to make sure it fits right before we pay for it. Three o'clock sound okay to you?"

I stifled a groan. "Yeah," I said, forcing a cheerful tone into my voice. Just the thought of the Barbie-pink nightmare made me want to shove a box of peanut butter M&M's into my mouth. "I'll be ready then."

"Great!" she squealed. "I can't wait to see it!"

The door shut in the aftermath of her excitement.

"Yeah," I muttered, grimacing. "Me too."

Chapter 46—The Best Wedding Gift

"**OMG LEXIE!** IT'S PERFECT!"

Kenzie's squeal carried through the bridal store when I stepped out of the dressing room in a monstrous pink horror. I waded forward, through the miles of fabric.

"Except through the shoulders . . . and the waist." Mom said, plucking at the dress with two fingers. "And the chest."

I'd avoided looking in the mirror of the dressing room out of sheer desperation and hope that I was still in a nightmare and would soon wake up, but no such luck. The hot pink terror was even more pink than I remembered, if possible.

"It will match the cake perfectly," Kenzie declared with smug triumph.

"Kenzie, it's at least three sizes too big now," Mom said.

"Nah, they can take it in at the seams."

The woman working in the store cleared her throat. "Um, actually, I think it *is* too big," she said. "We could take it in a little, but—"

Kenzie's eyes widened in instant panic. While Mom sought to soothe Kenzie's ruffled nerves, I snuck a glance past all of them to the three mirrors waiting against the wall and found exactly what I expected. A fluffy flamingo. The dress hung off me like a pair of old drapes, gowning my arms and torso in pink chiffon. Seeing Bradley while wearing such a hideous gown would surely cement my place in second-date-hell.

"Can you order the right size?" Kenzie asked the store worker, pulling me out of my thoughts. "We're two months away. That's plenty of time, right? Right?"

"Let me check," the store worker said, but the tug in her voice wasn't encouraging. She left with all too much eagerness to get away. Kenz had a hand in her hair, making her bangs stand straight up. Mom moved the fabric around my waist, folding it and playing with it, but it didn't make it any less of a monstrosity. I turned around to face my sister, the miles of fabric rustling around my legs as I moved.

"Kenz, I'm sorry."

"I knew you looked good," she said, "but I didn't realize you'd lost so much weight."

I'd been in the *Health and Happiness Society* for nearly four months and hadn't weighed in weeks. I didn't even know how much I had lost. I just knew that I felt better than I ever had in my life, and I'd just made an already appalling dress that much worse.

Maybe they won't have it in another size and I won't have to wear it, I thought with a glimmer of hope.

"No worries!" the bridal store worker chirped, returning with another dress the same color. "We have it in a smaller size. Let's give it a shot."

Kenzie clapped.

The bridal store worker slipped into the dressing room to help me, making me worry that we'd be stuffing my arms and torso into the dress. But it slid on with surprising ease, and I barely had to suck in while she zipped up the back. It did look better once it fit, but it was far from a great dress.

"Perfect," she said with a chipper smile. "I guess your dress size is a twelve now."

I whirled around. "What? What did you say?"

"This is a twelve. Your last dress was an eighteen."

"I've lost three dress sizes?"

She beamed. "Congrats!"

"But that doesn't make sense. I definitely can't fit into a size twelve pants. I just barely fit inside a size fourteen pair of pants and—"

She waved it off. "Dress sizes often fit differently and don't always reflect your pant size. Anyway, you should be proud of yourself. You've obviously worked very hard. And just in time for summer! June is only two weeks away. What a fun summer you will have!"

I stared in the mirror while she wafted out of the room, declaring, "It fits!" as she went. I could hardly believe it. *Size twelve.* Even if it wasn't my pant size, it didn't matter. I, Lexie Greene, fit into a size twelve. While it didn't feel as good as the day before when I finally submitted my story to the contest, it still felt *awesome.*

"Lexieeeee!" Kenzie called. "Hurry up. I want to see!"

With a resigned sigh and a promise to celebrate privately later, I slipped out of the dressing room. Kenz hopped up and down.

"AH!"

"It's very flattering," Mom said with a pleased smile.

Had she lost her mind? The flared skirt, the ruffled shoulders, and the massive bow around the waist was anything but flattering, although I wisely kept my opinions to myself. How could anyone find this appealing? Kenzie fluttered around like a little fairy, cooing over it. "Just look at the sash, and the ruffle! Ah! I love it even more than I did before."

"I have to wear it all day?"

"Yes! It will look lovely with the wedding cake and the decorations and your hair done up and makeup on and—"

Mom put a hand on Kenzie's shoulder and forced her to sit. "Calm down, Kenzie. You need to take a breath."

The temptation to make an excuse to leave overwhelmed me. This dress was miserable and would be hot in the middle of July. Everyone would think I was trying to dress up like Barbie or a pretty, pretty princess. But McKenzie looked so happy, and my mom so relieved, that I forced a smile.

"It's going to look great, Kenz," I said. "Really."

She clasped her hands and bit her bottom lip. "I know! I've never been so excited in my life! I already have big plans for your hair and makeup. We can get a Starbucks and go to my friend's house and get our hair and makeup done together that morning. It will be so much fun! And PEDICURES!! We can get pedicures together!"

Despite the inherent misery that would surely come with *playing dress up* with McKenzie for her wedding, I couldn't let her down on the big day just because it wasn't my definition of a good time. Kenzie wasn't perfect, and neither was our relationship, but we were closer than we'd ever been in our lives. I didn't want to break what Zumba had carefully built.

"Sounds great. I have that whole week dedicated to you."

Her eyes widened. "Really? I mean . . . you want to get pedicures? And do hair together? And . . . you'll go with me to try different styles of makeup?"

"Of course! My little sister is getting married, isn't she?" To my surprise, a clog of tears rose in my throat. "Besides, Dad would want us to do everything that a bride deserves for your big day, so let's go all out."

Whether it was the pool of tears in my eyes, or the moisture that came to Mom's, it must have been infectious because Kenz teared up instantly. She hopped up onto the platform and threw her arms around me.

"Thank you, Lexie! Thank you! Spending the day with you is the best wedding gift I could ask for."

I held her close, surprised at how fragile and small she felt. Kenzie and I had always lived on opposite sides of our family track, and now I wondered how much of that was my fault. Hadn't I just been too intimidated by, or jealous of, her pixie-like body and happy demeanor? I squeezed her extra tight.

"I love you, Kenz, and I'm so excited for you. You'll be the most beautiful bride."

"You're the best sister," she cried. "The best!"

I certainly hadn't been *the best sister* in the past, but now we had nothing but the future, and I knew it would be bright. I didn't have to be jealous or intimidated by Kenzie. A tear streaked down one side of Mom's face. Her lips trembled. I held out one arm.

"Come on, Mom," I said. "Family hug."

Mom rushed forward and dissolved into tears as we enveloped her into our broken—but healing—little family.

Chapter 47—Not a Loss

"**Welcome to the fifth month** of the *Health and Happiness Society*, ladies. Congrats. How are you feeling?"

Bitsy stared expectantly at Mira and me, her hair brushed into a ponytail and eyebrows raised. She wore the usual set of gym pants and oversized shirt, only now the shirt was *really* oversized. I didn't know how much weight Bitsy had lost, but she looked phenomenal. Mira raised her hand—were we in third grade?—and Bitsy called on her.

"I feel like I have more energy, lately," Mira said. "I slipped back into my Pepsi addiction for a few weeks, but I recently talked myself out of it again, and now I feel better."

Bitsy nodded. "I'm proud of you for pulling away from it again. I'm sure that wasn't easy. As a side note, you're really toning up, Mira. We're going to have to repurpose all your muumuus soon. My daughters could use some new drapes."

I shot Mira a glance with a silent agreement. The tropical muumuus had to go and not just because they were many sizes too large now. Mira blushed but smiled with unbridled delight.

"How about you, Lexie?" Bitsy asked. "How are you feeling? It's the second week of June already and your sister's wedding fast approaches. Ready for it?"

Not to mention my deadline for the editing internship application, I thought.

"I feel like my weight loss has slowed," I said. "It doesn't seem to be as easy anymore. My pants aren't becoming as loose as fast as they used to, although working out is getting easier."

Bitsy smirked. "The farther you go, the more difficult it is. Doesn't it suck? When was the last time you weighed in?"

"Last month."

She smiled in a conspiratorial kind of way. "Aren't you the least bit curious?"

My heart sped up in nervous energy for just a second. I thought of my nightly phone conversations with Bradley, of going out to breakfast with Rachelle the day before and not even wanting to eat Krispy Kremes. I'd just run two miles for the first time earlier in the week, so I was still progressing. Did it matter what I weighed anymore?

"No," I said, surprising more than just myself. "It doesn't really matter, does it?"

She smiled. "Not if you feel like it doesn't."

Mira reached over and squeezed my hand with a warm smile.

"Neither of you ate, right?" Bitsy asked, shunting the conversation back to business. "You both got my text? Good. Because I'm about to blow your mind with the best, most nutritious meal ever. Green smoothies!"

Bitsy grabbed a blender she'd displayed on her kitchen counter where the three of us congregated. A display of various fruits and veggies littered the counter top, as well as small cups for sampling. "For those of you who hate veggies, this could save your life. I'm about to show you how to hide spinach. Not even my girls notice it."

Bitsy reached for a bottle of something labeled kefir—whatever black magic that was—and dumped a small portion into the clean blender. Her kitchen was so sparkly and pristine that I didn't even lean against the counter, worried I'd smudge something and have to pay a penance of push-ups. While Bitsy passed around a printout of smoothie recipes to *supercharge your morning energy*, my cell phone went off, and I reached into my backpack.

Miss Bliss.

"Keep going," I told Bitsy while holding up my phone. "I just need to take this call."

I stepped onto Bitsy's porch where hanging flower baskets dripped with flowers of bright purple and pink. The once cool spring air had started to warm, leaving a sticky haze behind. My flip-flops and shorts—which I'd never worn in public before—kept my still cottage-cheesy-and-less-than-perfect legs cool.

"Hello?"

"Lexie, it's Miss Bliss. I'm calling with news on your story."

I sat on the top step of the porch, but still held onto the railing. "Okay."

"Not sure why they notified me instead of you," she said, smacking an obnoxious wad of gum. "Must be because I'm your advisor or something, but you didn't get it. You didn't win."

"I didn't?"

"No. I can't figure out why, either. I'm not sure who *did* win, but I'm bugged enough that it wasn't yours, let me tell you."

A feeling of devastation rolled through me. I'd put my heart and soul into that piece. I'd worked on it for weeks on end, barely emerging from a writing-induced-haze to finish it for the final competition. I was supposed to win! My life had been going so well. I'd been on a fairytale roll for a while.

Ice cream, I thought, barraged with thoughts of sugar and cream and the sweet taste of it on a hot summer day. *I'd feel better with ice cream.*

"I see," I said when the silence stretched too long. "Well, that's a definite disappointment."

"Yeah," she muttered. "They sure took long enough to decide, didn't they? Anyway, at this point I'd just suggest turning your application for the internship in."

"I will. I'll do that tonight."

"Great." She popped her gum, which seemed twice as loud through the phone. "Listen, Lex, I'm really sorry. I thought you had it. Your story is . . . wonderful. Just because one crummy competition doesn't pick you up doesn't mean it's not a great story."

Moose Tracks or Mint Chocolate Chip. Or a hot fudge sundae.

"Yeah."

Miss Bliss rattled off a few other things, but they barely registered. I mumbled a response and finally hung up as soon as she did. The quiet of Bitsy's idyllic, sweet neighborhood followed in the aftermath.

Yep. Definitely could use some ice cream.

"Bad news?"

Mira's voice came from behind me seconds before she sat on the top stair at my side. Bitsy flanked me on the right, bearing a small cup with a pink, blended confection inside.

"Disappointing news," I countered. Bad news was Dad dying. "My story didn't win that big competition."

"Oh," Mira said, putting her hand on my back. "That's so disappointing, Lexie. You worked hard on that story."

"Here," Bitsy said. "Have a strawberry smoothie with kefir. It has a lot of probiotics."

I snorted out an amused laugh. "Thanks."

"So what now?" Mira asked.

"I submit my application without having had a winning entry to pad it and then hope for the best. There's not much more I can do, really."

"Are you going to be okay?" Bitsy asked, searching my face.

"I'm sad," I admitted. "I wanted to win."

"But is that why you wrote that story? I mean, of all the stories in your head that you could have written, did you write that one just to win?"

Her question stopped me in my tracks. I'd written that story as a way of soul-searching, of finding Lexie Greene and coming to terms with my past.

"No. I didn't write it just for the competition."

"Then it's not a loss."

"You've seemed happier than I've ever seen you ever since you finished that story," Mira said. "It's like you came into yourself."

"Or started the journey of *accepting* yourself, flaws and all." Bitsy wrapped her arms around her legs. "It's not an easy one, heaven knows."

"Yeah," I said, finding a smile. "I guess you're right."

Bitsy nodded to the cup in my hand. "Drink your smoothie. It's okay to be disappointed you didn't win, just find a way to cope with it outside of Rocky Road, okay?"

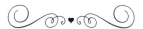

I kept a firm grip on the steering wheel the whole drive home to stop myself from making an unnecessary detour to Burger King for one of their cheap ice cream cones.

Instead of holing up in my basement lair, I took my laptop upstairs and sat at the kitchen table. Mom bustled around the house, talking to herself in random spurts. She hummed as she watered the flowers, or called up questions to Kenzie about the wedding. It had been a long time since I'd involved myself in the daily movement of life above ground, and I found it warmer than the quiet of my basement lair.

I stared at a full application screen, reviewed every line twice, attached the requisite essay that Miss Bliss had already proofread, and hit the *submit* button. For being something I'd thought about so much lately, in the end, the process was very anticlimactic. But wasn't that just life? I seemed to always build up expectations that never flushed themselves out entirely.

Just like watching my weight on the scale, what I learned in the journey of accomplishing my goal was far more important than hitting a certain weight or winning a competition. I'd never really written that story to win, or for Miss Bliss, or for Bradley.

I'd written it for me, and that was enough.

The sound of Mom running water into a saucepan drew me out of my reverie. "Hey, Mom," I said, closing my laptop. "Need some help fixing dinner?"

Chapter 48—Freak Out

The morning of Kenzie's wedding dawned without regard to the fact that I hadn't gone to bed yet.

Amidst the mess of cleaning the house in case of last-minute guests, ensuring the table decorations were done, the bouquets safe in the fridge, the groom's family escorted to the hotel, and Kenzie properly stressed out over the status of her hairdresser, sleep eluded both Mom and I. I tossed the final name card onto the appropriate pile and slouched back in the kitchen chair.

"I didn't know it was possible to be this tired."

"Oh, Lexie," Mom said, rubbing a hand over her face. "I forgot to have you try your dress on. I hung it in your closet downstairs. Go make sure it fits."

I yawned. "We already know it's going to fit. I tried it on weeks ago."

"Just go put it on. If you don't, Kenzie's going to ask about it. If you've already tried it on, we can tell her that it looks great, and it'll save some time in between the mani-pedi, the hair dresser, and getting her dress on within the next six hours."

Her head fell to her folded arms when the grandfather clock in the front room tolled six times. I groaned. "I need an energy drink."

"I'll grab some coffee or something," Mom said wearily. "At least Kenzie got some sleep last night. She's the one that's the most important today. We'll sleep later, okay?"

Yeah, I thought, *she slept because I secretly drugged her with Benadryl at ten.*

Rachelle breezed into the house just as I'd convinced myself, and my exhausted feet, to stand.

"I'm here, Lex. And I brought breakfast!" She sailed into the kitchen with a box of doughnuts. "Don't worry. I found an egg white omelet for you, and doughnuts for the rest of . . . well . . . whoever. I came to see if there's anything I can help with last minute."

"Thanks, Rachelle," Mom said, patting her on the shoulder as she walked past. "I'm going to go shower and wake myself up a bit. I think we just finished the last-minute preparations."

Rachelle gave me a once over. "You look like death."

"C'mon," I said. "You can help me into the monster."

She clapped and hopped to the basement door. "The flamingo monstrosity?" she squealed. "I can't wait to finally see it!"

Ten minutes—and an epic struggle with an unholy amount of material—later, I stood in front of my bathroom mirror with a pale face and wide eyes.

Oh no.

"Your sister is going to freak out, Lexie."

Rachelle stared at me in the mirror, her eyes wide, jaw slack. I mirrored her expression of horror with one of my own. The ridiculous pink bridesmaid dress was, once again, too big. Although not as dramatic as last time, the neckline hung slack and the waist drooped. Kenzie's wedding was less than six hours away, and my dress looked like I'd picked it off the floor without regard to size.

"I thought I'd be able to maintain," I cried, pressing my palms to my flushed cheeks. "I didn't think I was losing enough weight to cause the dress to look horrible. My weight loss has seemed so slow! She's going to kill me!"

Rachelle pulled the waist out an inch. "Well, it was over a month ago when you last tried it on, right?"

"I . . . I suppose so."

She grinned. "Oh man, Lexie. This is the best thing ever. No way she's going to let you wear this! You're off the hook. You're free. You won't have to wear the flamingo monstrosity!"

"No, Rachelle, you don't get it. Kenzie's going to be furious! I'm the maid of honor. I have to wear pink. I have some safety pins in the top drawer. Fix this. Now."

"Okay, okay. It'll be fine. Kenzie isn't even going to notice. We'll just dress you at the last possible moment and everything will be great. She'll be so focused on getting married that she won't be thinking of her maid of honor."

Her soothing reassurance didn't reassure me at all. My cell phone dinged, signaling a text message. I snatched it off the desk.

Bradley.

Hey! Tell me when and where I'm supposed to be, and I'll be there. Just crashed at my friend's new house last night.

My stomach fluttered. How had I almost forgotten that I'd be seeing Bradley again?

At this point, I think it'll be best to meet you at the venue.

Too easy, he immediately replied. *You emailed me the information already, right?*

Yes.

See you then. Let me know if I can help.

Rachelle accidentally poked me in the back with a safety pin.

"Ow!"

"Sorry. I'm trying to figure out if we can pull this waist in so it doesn't look so flabby."

Ten minutes of experimentation later, the dress appeared to fit better, but lacked symmetry. "It looks like my left boob is . . . funky. Can you see the safety pins? What about my neckline? It's higher on one side."

"Well . . . not exactly. Look, it's fine. No one is going to notice. They'll be staring at Kenzie."

"Rachelle! This isn't going to work!"

"Lexie!" Kenzie called from the top of the stairs. "We need to leave for the nail place in five minutes!"

"Be right there!" I turned to Rachelle in a half-panic. "Please take it to Mira and have her take it in a little? She can sew, maybe she can work some magic. Just don't say a word about it to anyone! Not even Mom. She can't handle anything else, and she'll break down into a crying fit that I'm not prepared to handle. Sneak it out of here, okay?"

Despite the massive amount of material in the dress, she didn't even act concerned. "Sure," she said immediately. "No problem."

The dress rustled as I pulled it over my head, and then a loud ripping sound tore through the air. My stomach lurched.

"Rachelle?" I whispered from the midst of material. She swore under her breath.

"Don't move, Lexie. Just let me work it off you."

Bit by bit she carefully pulled the dress off me. Once free, I looked up in horror to find the left sleeve dangling by a few pink strings.

"No!"

"It's all right," Rachelle said, rolling the dress over her arm. "I got this. It'll be fine, Lex. Don't worry about it. Mira and I will fix everything. I promise. Go have fun with your sister."

"This is a nightmare."

"Nope, we're good."

"LEXIE!" Kenzie called. "We have to go *now!*"

"Coming!"

I threw myself into a pair of jeans, flip-flops, and a black shirt. "Are you sure?"

Rachelle waved me away. "Go! I'll take care of it. I'll meet you at the bridal room at the venue in three hours. It's going to be fine."

I slipped my phone into my back pocket, grabbed my purse, and hurried up the stairs two at a time. "Sorry Kenz!" I cried, forcing a fake smile on my face when I made it to the top. "I was just making sure the dress fit. Let's go!"

Kenzie stood in a pair of shorts, a button up shirt and a similar pair of flip-flops. Despite it being her happy day, a slight glaze of panic covered her eyes that I'd seen for the past 72 hours of finalizing wedding preparations.

"Is it okay?" she asked. "It fits, right? It's going to look great?"

"Beautiful!" I cried, grabbing her by the shoulder. "Let's get going. It's time to get you ready for the wedding."

Chapter 49—Maid of Honor

"**Can we make** my hairstyle subtle?" I asked the hairdresser, a middle-aged black woman named Terry with an impressive row of white teeth. "I don't want anything flashy or bright. Please don't match my eye shadow with the dresses?"

"Yeah," she agreed, her upper lip curling slightly. "Flashy wouldn't look good on you. How about we straighten your hair and add a few curls? I'll go easy on the makeup too, although I think we need to at least try fake lashes."

"Fake lashes? They *have* those?"

Terry rolled her eyes. "Girl, have you been living under a rock? They're fabulous. Just trust me. You're in good hands."

I blew out a long breath. "Okay."

Kenzie and Mom sat to my left, chattering. Outside, a bank of dark clouds rolled in from the west with occasional low growls and the threat of rain. Thankfully, we were safely tucked in the bridal suite at the venue, preparing for the indoor ceremony.

My eyes strayed to the clock on the wall while Terry went to work tugging and pulling on my head. Two hours left. My fingers and toes sparkled with new nails in a horrid shade of pink that matched every other horrid decoration. The other bridesmaids would start trickling in soon. All eight of them.

My phone buzzed and I flipped it over so quickly it nearly clattered to the floor. I bobbled with it for a second before catching it in a firm grasp.

"Nervous?" Terry asked, brandishing a blow dryer like a gun, one eyebrow raised.

"Just expecting a text."

Mira and I have it under control, Rachelle's message said, *but it's going to take at least an hour.*

Although I wouldn't really relax until I could see the dress myself, a surge of relief moved through me. Mira would make it work. She could do anything. Terry worked in silence while I fiddled with my

210

phone, inserted comments into the conversation when Kenzie asked me a question, and worried, in general, over the possibly disastrous wedding. Would the dress fit? Would Bradley like it?

An hour later, Terry stepped back, smirking.

"Mmm hmm," she murmured. "Just as I thought."

Kenzie, who had just finished with her own hair dresser, stood up. Her mouth went slack and eyes wide.

"Wow. Lexie?"

"What?"

"I hardly even recognize you. You're gorgeous."

Because of my struggling relationship with mirrors, I'd studiously avoided the awkwardness of staring at myself for sixty minutes.

"Go on," Terry said with a chuckle. "See if you like it."

When I first looked up, I didn't see Lexie Greene. In fact, I looked at several places in the mirror just to make sure that the girl I stared at was actually me. My hair, usually in a ponytail or limp on my shoulders, fell in wide, gentle curls around a thinner face. I could actually see cheekbones. Terry had somehow wrangled fake eyelashes onto my eyes, which made them both dark and bright at the same time.

"Oh," I said. "Oh."

Mom rustled up to my side, half in her new dress, half out, her hair coiffed into a fashionable bun that suited a mother-of-the-bride.

"Lexie! You look wonderful."

I touched the tips of my silky hair, thinking about Bradley and how he would react. *Perfect,* I thought. *This is exactly what I wanted to look like for him. Maybe this won't be so bad after all.*

"Thank you, Terry. It's perfect."

She snorted. "I know."

The door to the bridal suite popped open, bringing a sweeping current of wind into the room.

"Hello bridal party!" Mira called, walking—not toddling—in with a long bag draped over her left arm. "Kenzie, look at you! You're ravishing. Yes, just beautiful. Anyway, no time to chat, Rachelle and I need to get ready but we've had a little problem with Lexie's dress."

"Nothing big." Rachelle tried to wave it off but her smile faltered. "It's just that the sleeve tore and it's too big and—"

"Kenzie, baby, it's hideous on her," Mira said. "Besides, the maid of honor is special, so they normally have a different dress than the other bridesmaids. I couldn't salvage the pink one, to be honest. It wasn't a very well made dress in the first place. No, no, don't cry. Aunty Mira has saved the day."

She shucked the long bag on her arm off, revealing a simple black dress, elegant, but classy, that was almost the same style as the pink horror, minus the obnoxious bow in front. I held my breath, hardly daring to hope. Would Kenzie let it happen?

"Your wedding colors are black and pink, right?" Mira continued easily, not giving Kenzie a chance to respond. "Well, we found a black dress in Lexie's size, and we bought a pink sash that matches the other bridesmaid dresses to go with it. It's going to look beautiful."

"But it's different," Kenzie whispered, eyes watering. "I wanted pink!"

"Well, technically it's more *in fashion* this way," Rachelle said. "Most brides have a different dress to distinguish the maid of honor."

I'd seen that expression on Rachelle's face before. Tight jaw, twitching lips. She was lying through her teeth, and I loved her for it.

"Really?" Kenzie asked, her brows wrinkled.

Mira nodded to drive the point home. "Really, Kenz. I think this is best. And, to be honest, it's your only option. The other dress would have looked terrible and the sleeve is torn."

Kenzie ran her eyes over the black dress and let out a long breath. "Okay, I guess. If that's the only option. You're sure?"

Mira nodded.

As if summoned on cue, the door slammed open again, spilling five of Kenzie's friends into the room at the same time. They swooped on the bride like a flock of overripe flamingos, squealing and oohing until I could hardly stand it. I grabbed Rachelle and Mira and pulled them off to the side.

"Thank you! How can I ever repay you?"

"Lexie, I didn't want to say anything in front of your sister since this is her big day, but you're absolutely stunning," Mira cried, inspecting my face and hair. "I just know you're going to knock Bradley's socks off in this dress. Rachelle and I have been practicing how we were going to convince Kenzie the whole way here. I'm so relieved it worked!"

"Truly," Rachelle agreed with a similar grin. "You're perfection today. Let's get you into it. Mira and I have to go change and get ready. We've been at five different bridal stores trying to find a dress that would work. It's a miracle we got it at all. What time is it? I can't tell, my phone battery just died."

"We have just under an hour before the ceremony," I said, checking my own phone. "Let's get this done and make sure it fits."

Ten minutes later I stepped out of a changing room and stood before a three-way mirror. The black dress, svelte and slenderizing, fit me like a dream. I ran my palm along the smooth front panel, giving me an hourglass figure that I'd never had before. My hips were still plentiful, and my chest as well, but I no longer looked like a bowling ball with arms and legs. No. I looked, and felt, like a beautiful woman.

Something I'd never experienced before.

"It's perfect," I said, throwing my arms around Mira. "Thank you!"

"We have to go." Rachelle tugged Mira's sleeve. "Like *now*. If not we'll miss the ceremony."

"Oh, dear. Yes. Lexie, we'll see you afterwards."

They bustled out, leaving me to watch the chattering hoard of friends, who had already wrangled Kenz into her dress. A peal of thunder cracked the sky. Mom rushed over to me five minutes later in pure panic.

"Lexie! Where's Mira? I just called her but she's not answering. I need her now!"

"Gone. What's wrong?"

Mom pressed her hands to her face. "I left the picture of your father at home! The one that Kenzie insists be on the chair next to me during the ceremony. We can't do the wedding without him. We can't. She'll kill me!"

I grabbed my phone to call Rachelle, but stopped. "Rachelle's battery is dead. Is there anyone that can stop by the house and pick it up?"

"It's locked."

"Fine, I'll go," I said, grabbing my car keys. "Just stay here with Kenzie and she'll never even know, okay? I'll be right back. Stay calm. I'll be gone twenty minutes."

Mom's hands fluttered nervously over her chest. "Okay. Calm."

The wind rustled my hair when I hurried to the car, barefoot because I didn't want to get my ultra-bright pink flip-flops dirty and risk breaking down the last of Kenzie's fragile guards. By the time I made it to the house, raindrops pattered lightly on my head.

"No," I growled, yanking the front door open. "Don't rain until I get back!"

Dad's picture, a beautifully framed photo of him a few months before his death, waited on the table. I snatched it, caught one last delighted look at myself in the mirror, and rushed back to the car. As if the gods of rain wanted to mock me, the clouds split open, and an instant flood descended. By the time I drove down the street, a deluge obstructed my vision. A loud honking noise startled me from my thoughts two seconds before a pair of headlights skidded through an intersection and slammed into the back of my car.

♥
Chapter 50—Lexie, Shut Up.
♠

For about ten seconds, all I could do was stare at my rearview mirror and the rain pounding my cracked back window. Had that just happened?

You've got to be kidding me.

"No!" I groaned. "Not *now*! Kenzie is going to kill me!"

Smoke billowed out of the hood of the other car, and fearing for their life, I ejected my seat belt and threw my door open. An elderly woman sat in the driver's seat, staring blankly at her steering wheel. I rushed up to her window, rain pounding my shoulders and hair.

"Are you okay?" I asked. She blinked, in a daze. I jerked open her door. "Ma'am? Are you all right? Do you need me to call an ambulance?"

"I-I'm fine," she said, rubbing her chest where the seatbelt crossed her ribs. "Just . . . a bit disoriented."

Her airbag had deployed, leaving an acrid scent behind and bitter powder in the air. Although smoke continued to plume and hiss from her car, I didn't see any flames.

"Are you having a hard time breathing?"

"No. I'm . . . I'm fine."

"I'm going to call the police," I said. "You stay here."

She nodded weakly and I shut the door before the deluge soaked her skinny, frail little body. By the time I made it back to my car, water had seeped through my dress. The warm chill pressed against my skin when I climbed back inside, grabbed my cell, and called 911. Rain fell so hard I could barely read the street sign across the road to tell them where to come. Once I finished reporting the accident, I slipped back outside.

"That's all I need," I muttered, jogging through the rain soaked grass in my bare feet, "is some sweet old lady to have a heart attack or something."

I knocked on her window. She shook her head and cracked open the door. The haze of shock had started to retreat from her glazed eyes.

"The police are on the way," I said. "Are you sure you're okay? Do you want me to have them send the ambulance?"

"No," she said weakly. "No, I'm fine. I just . . . I lost control. It's like the water just carried my car, and I'm . . . oh goodness, I'm so sorry! I really didn't mean to hit you. It was an accident. And your dress will be ruined. Just an accident, I swear!"

Tears welled up in her old eyes. She held out a shaky hand for me. I took it and gave an affectionate little squeeze to reassure her. My dress was the least of my worries now. Water streaked down the side of my head in long rivulets.

"Don't worry," I said. "I'm not angry. Accidents happen. I'm just glad you're feeling all right."

Not wanting to soak her, I retreated to wait in my car until the police arrived. Attempts to call Mom were futile. She likely didn't hear her phone over the cacophony of Kenzie's friends and last-minute preparations. Mira and Rachelle were also MIA. A mild state of panic started in my chest. I had to get to the wedding! How was I going to get there if no one answered? Would they wait? Would Kenzie freak out? My phone chimed with a text.

Hey, Bradley had written. *Just got here. Will I be able to see you beforehand?*

My heart skipped a beat. Bradley! I hit the *send* button to call him and pressed the phone to my rain-saturated face. He answered after one ring.

"Hey, girl."

"Bradley!" I cried. "Oh, I'm so glad you answered. I need help. I was just in a car accident, and no one is answering their phone, and I need a ride and—"

"Whoa, whoa. Are you all right?"

"Yeah, yeah. Just some sweet old lady hit me. Please come get me?"

"Of course." The sound of shuffling and car keys rang in the background. "I'm on it. Where are you?"

I gave him a quick set of directions just as the whirling red and blue lights of a police car drove up. After making sure Bradley knew how to find me, I stepped back into the deluge just as the police officer stepped out of his car.

"You all right?" he asked. I nodded, pointing to the Cadillac that belched steam.

"There's an old lady in that car. Says she's fine."

He motioned for me to wait there, spoke with the woman for a minute, and came back to my side while opening an umbrella. By the time I'd explained what had happened, a familiar junky car pulled up across the street. My throat tightened.

NO! I told myself. *You will not cry. You will not cry.*

"Lex! You okay?"

Bradley jogged to my side, taking my breath away in a white shirt, tie, and black pants that could have used a pass or two with the iron. His hair was slightly ruffled as though he'd forgotten to brush it, but he still looked adorable and strong and everything I had imagined he would be. My stomach twisted into a series of knots. A trickle of rain rushed down my back in a long stream.

"I'm fine," I said, though my hands had started to tremble a bit. "I'm fine."

He put his arm around my shoulders and pulled me close. I wanted to melt into his comforting strength, the instant warmth of his broad shoulders. "Can she wait in the car, officer? She's soaked and needs to get to a wedding."

The officer nodded, motioning with a jerk of his head. Bradley led me back to the driver's seat and helped me inside. I caught a glimpse of myself in the rearview mirror with a gasp of horror. My hair hung limp and wet, not unlike a drowned rat, around my shoulders. One of Terry's carefully placed fake eyelashes had come unglued on one end and flapped around my eye. Mascara and eyeliner streaked my pasty white face, making me look like a gothic clown. By the time Bradley ran around and slipped in the passenger seat, I couldn't stop the hot tears filling my eyes.

"Girl, are you sure you're okay?" he asked, his shoulders wet from the rain. "You didn't get whiplash or hurt or something did you? Do you need an ambulance?"

"It's ruined!" I cried, putting my face into my hands and leaning into the steering wheel. "Everything is ruined."

"What's ruined?"

"This perfect day!"

"We'll get you to the wedding, don't worry. The officer is filling out paperwork now."

"No!" I wailed. "I didn't mean that, but that's awful too! I just . . . I . . . I wanted everything to be perfect when I saw you again. My hair was done and so was my makeup and for the first time in my life I looked and felt beautiful, instead of feeling fat and sorry for myself. I even wore a black dress just like I had always dreamed! Now I look like I just drowned in the river, and they had to dredge my body from the bottom. And I know that looks aren't everything and neither is size or the scale, but I still wanted to be beautiful and perfect and . . . and I'm still not perfect now, and it doesn't even matter because it's all ruined!"

The last of my confession came out in a keening cry, and I gave into a pathetic little sob. Despite all I had learned from Megan, from myself, from the *Health and Happiness Society*, I still felt a burning need for Bradley to like me back. It compounded my self-frustration, and I cried even harder.

At first I thought I surely heard wrong, but the sound of Bradley laughing soon had my cries stuttering to a stop. I peeked out between my fingers and the hot tears gliding down them.

"What?" I asked, sniffling back snot before it, too, covered my face. "What's so funny?"

Bradley had tipped his head back as he released full belly-laughs. "I think you're insane," he finally managed to say.

"You think I'm—"

"You thought you weren't beautiful or perfect?" His murky hazel eyes narrowed. "Lexie, you're the most beautiful, perfect girl that I've ever met."

I stared at him, certain that I'd hit my head in the accident and was now hallucinating.

"What? But I'm . . . I'm a bigger girl."

He turned to the side and leaned a shoulder against the back of the seat so he could face me. "Lexie, I don't care if you're a size zero or thirty-four—I think you're perfect."

"Perfect? Are you kidding? I have hips and—"

"Yeah, and I have big shoulders." He shrugged. "So what?"

"So," I whispered. "Your shoulders are attractive, at least."

"So are your hips."

My heart beat so hard in my chest I could feel the blood course all the way into the tips of my fingers. It all seemed so unreal. He actually liked my curvy figure? As in . . . that could happen? Since when were hips attractive? "Really?"

"Really. They're a part of you, and it's you that I like."

He reached over and put a hand under my chin. "Don't ever think that you have to wear makeup or lose weight or fix your hair to be good enough for me. If anyone should be trying to match up, it's me trying to be worthy of you. Lexie, I had to borrow a pair of pants from my friend because I forgot them. I drive a car that was made before I was born. And I don't have the heart or determination that you do. So maybe I should be the one worried that this is all going to go wrong."

"No, no, no," I said. "You have it all wrong."

"Lexie, shut up. You're beautiful and perfect, even if your makeup is streaked, and your hair is wet, and your dress is ruined. I've never been more attracted to you than I am right now."

Tears pooled in my eyes again. I swallowed. "Thank you," I whispered.

"I'm going to go check with the cop to see what he says. You stay in here, I'll be right back. We need to get you to that wedding."

Chapter 51—My Story

Ten minutes before the ceremony was supposed to start, I rushed into the bridal suite completely drenched but holding Dad's photo safely in my arms. One of my fake eyelashes still hung from my eye, flapping every time I blinked.

"LEXIE!" The shriek came from Kenzie, swathed in all white. One of the bridesmaids stood at her side, swatting her hand away every time Kenzie tried to gnaw on her perfectly manicured nails. "WHERE HAVE YOU BEEN? And . . . wait . . . what happened to you?"

Mom rushed forward. "What happened?"

"I got in a car accident," I said, passing the photo off to Mom. "I was on my way back from getting Dad's picture. Some old lady hydroplaned and ran into me. Look, that doesn't matter right now. I've already called Terry. She's on her way over to fix . . . this."

I waved a hand over my hair, catching sight of myself in the mirror with a cringe.

"An accident?" Kenzie cried. "Are you all right? Are you hurt?"

"An accident?" Mom echoed, and both rushed forward to flutter over me. "Are you okay? Why didn't you call? What happened? I knew I shouldn't have sent you!"

"I'm fine, I'm fine," I said, batting them off. "I'll go over the details later."

"Is anyone hurt?"

"No, no, it's fine. Can we delay the ceremony for just a few minutes so I can clean up?"

Kenz nodded. "Of course, Lex. As long as you're okay. I'm . . . are you sure? You don't have to stand up there."

I smiled. "No, I'm definitely going to be there for my little sister's wedding. I just hope you don't mind me standing in a puddle."

Mom, seeing that I wasn't about to die a horrible death, sprang into action. "I'll let the venue know. They'll make an announcement that there's been a delay. Yes, an announcement. That's what I'll do. Need to make an announcement."

She bustled away, having found a job to occupy her for the moment.

"I'm here!" Terry declared from the door, waving a hairdryer and a brush. "Get in a chair, Lex. Kenz, you stand back and look beautiful. Flock of flamingos, back off. Terry is in town now. We have a wedding to look fabulous for."

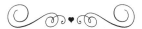

The wedding venue rained in flowers pink and black. Tulle swept the aisles, decorated the chairs, and filled the arbor that the pastor stood in front of. I recognized only a portion of the people that I passed while I walked down the aisle. Bradley sat in the back, looking burly, and a bit out of place with his rumpled hair, but handsome all the same.

Despite a twenty-minute delay while Terry straightened my hair, Mom blow-dried my dress, and one of the flamingos cleaned my face and reapplied a simple layer of makeup, every seat in the room was packed full. An organ played in the background, McKenzie sparkled, and Mom cried through the whole thing.

It was perfect.

Kenzie and her groom disappeared outside in a hailstorm of applause once it finished. I hung back, watching the milling crowd surge out the doors. The reception would immediately follow the ceremony in a different part of the venue. Bradley waited in his seat, then filtered through the crowd when the chaos died down.

"You look beautiful, girl." He smirked. "You certainly cleaned up fast."

I returned his grin with a wry smile of my own. My hair was straight and dry. No curls. Not much body. I wore only a simple slash of eyeliner and some mascara, but I didn't care. I felt great. Although I'd felt beautiful before, I felt like regular Lexie now, and it was regular Lexie that had something to say.

"Thanks. Hey, listen, I meant to tell you that Kenzie wants me to mill around for a while, talk to everyone. She said just for the first hour or so. We have family in town that I haven't seen since Dad died, so they all want to catch up. To spare you the agony of small talk, I brought something to occupy your time while I catch up with my crazy old aunts."

His eyebrows rose. "Oh really?"

I tugged his sleeve. "Really. Follow me."

We slipped out a side door before anyone noticed. Once in the bridal suite, now deserted and flamingo-free, I reached for my backpack and pulled out a thick stack of papers.

"Here," I said, extending it to him.

He grabbed it, eyes narrowed. "Is this what I think it is?"

"Depends on what you think it is."

"Your story."

My stomach fluttered. "Yes. It's the story that I submitted to the competition, except I added more to it. It's still not quite finished, but I wanted you to read it as it is now."

"*Bon Bons to Yoga Pants?*" he asked, reading the title with a quirked eyebrow.

I glanced down to the collection of papers and bit my bottom lip. Although I'd planned out exactly what I wanted to say before I handed my heart over to him in its inky entirety, the words failed me. I relied on the first thing that came to my mind.

"Yeah, *Bon Bons to Yoga Pants*. It's a story about a girl that used to eat bon bons all the time, and lived in fear of yoga pants because they were formfitting. It's . . . my story. Look, I think you probably won't care about my past, but it's important to me that you know and understand who I am. I mean . . . who I have been. Although I suppose that who I have been all these years has led to who I am now. Anyway . . . it's important to me. And," I added in a small voice. "You happen to be in it. A lot."

His lips twisted in a little smile, but he remained quiet. I pulled in a deep breath to gain a little strength. The words that I knew I needed to use stuck in my throat, but I forced them out.

"Bradley, I . . . I used to be very overweight."

The words came out with more velocity than I intended. Although I watched his eyes carefully, trying to detect any sign of horror or disgust, I saw nothing. He simply listened, waiting for me to finish. It gave me the strength to keep going.

"I mean it. I weighed in at 259 pounds at the beginning of this year. My dad died of a heart attack, and he had always been very sedentary and heavy as well. I kind of followed in his footsteps all my life. I hated myself. I never did anything healthy, and I turned to food when my problems scared me. But now I've . . . I've finally started to actually live. So when Miss Bliss told me to write about something raw and real and . . . well, *me*, I decided to tell my story."

I let out a long breath, having run out of steam, and felt suddenly exhausted.

"I guess that's it," I said, smiling sheepishly. "I just needed you to know who I really am before we figure out whether this is going to go anywhere. And, uh, don't get freaked out by . . . well, whatever you read about yourself."

Bradley fanned the pages then looked at me with a crooked smile. "Thanks."

Such a simple word, but it struck me to my heart. His beautiful murky eyes said everything else. I swallowed back my relief, feeling fifty pounds lighter.

"Yeah, sure. Anyway, I thought you could start reading it while I do the necessary mingling."

He held out his hand for me to take and grinned. "I'd love to read your story, Lexie Greene. Let's go. Your crowd awaits."

Chapter 52—It's Beautiful

Mingling took on a whole new meaning when applied to a crowd the size that Kenzie and her fiancé drew in.

Although I had to entertain family, engage in small talk, wave, laugh, joke, and reminisce, I kept an eye on Bradley. He sat at a circular table in the back, a glass of ice water and my book in front of him. From the moment he sat down, he hadn't taken his eyes away. I watched carefully in between swapping memories and thanking people for their support, silently wishing I could sneak away and apply a suction cup to Bradley's brain. I wanted to funnel all his thoughts so I knew exactly what he was thinking of me.

Was I good enough? Would he bail now that he knew the truth about my love affair with food and all my many imperfections? An hour and a half into the reception, I looked up to check on him and saw nothing but an empty table. My gut clenched.

What if he left?

I peeled myself away from old Uncle Bart with a smile and a promise to pull his finger later. The venue opened up onto an extensive set of gardens in the backyard, complete with a canopy of twinkle lights and green hedges interspersed with naked-angel fountains. A cool rush of air greeted me. The sky still remained overcast, though it hadn't rained again. I ventured forward down a stone path to the right to find a familiar set of broad shoulders staring at a mossy pond. Honeysuckle cloaked a trellis off to the side, and the tinkle of a fountain rang through the still air.

"Bradley?"

He looked up and smiled, hands tucked into his pants pocket. "Hey, girl."

"Is everything all right?" My shoes clacked as I walked, a strange background noise to the Sinatra music floating from the reception. The distant sound of glasses clinking and people murmuring in conversation filled the rest of the space. Despite the obvious presence of others inside, the ambiance made me feel oddly alone with him.

"Yeah, of course. I was just . . . thinking."

My breathing sped up of its own volition. I forced myself to calm down. "Is this where I offer a penny for your thoughts?"

He chuckled. "Nah. You can have my thoughts for free." He motioned to a rock nearby where my book sat. Over half the pages were folded back. "I was just thinking about your story."

I swallowed. "And?"

"I have two trains of thought so far. Want to hear them both?"

Do I? I wanted to ask back. "Of course."

His eyes narrowed on something in the distance. "I'm amazed that you don't see what I see. It's baffling that the confident, beautiful girl I've met, that I've always been a little intimidated by, doesn't realize how . . . I don't know . . . strong you are."

My mouth dropped open. "You've been intimidated by me?"

"Uh . . . yeah. Big time. By the way, I'm also obsessed with Arby's roast beef and curly fries, so I'm thinking that's where we need to go tonight." He gazed around. "Probably soon. The monster in my belly needs to be fed."

I smiled, startled to feel tears in my eyes. With concerted effort I blinked them away and forced an even tone. "And what's your second train of thought?"

"That you and I aren't so different. I'm more like you than you think. You've obviously had me on some sort pedestal that I don't deserve, which is frightening in itself." He cracked a smile, though I saw a hint of uncertainty behind it. "I'm not sure I'll be able to live up to your opinion of me, you know."

"I think you already have," I whispered.

"I think it's time for a dance." He held out a hand and I slipped mine inside his. His palm felt warm and smooth, sending bolts of heat through my arm. "But, in the interest of full disclosure, I'm a horrible dancer. So I need you to tell me where to put my hands. Then we'll shuffle around like it's high school and try to win the-most-awkward-couple-award."

I laughed and placed his hand on my waist. "Unless we have a few cardio beats going and a Zumba disco ball, I'm terrible at dancing also."

We moved into a comfortable, easy rhythm. His thick shoulders and strong arms seemed to engulf me. I'd never felt so safe in my life.

Several minutes passed while the chime of the reception continued in the background, leaving my thoughts to wander.

"Listen, Lex, I really like you." He pulled away just enough to look me in the eyes. "I want something to happen between us, and I'm ready to say *thumbs up let's do this*. But I'm going to be honest: I've always worried that I'm not good enough for someone as motivated and strong as you, and now I'm even more worried because I see how far you've come. Are you willing to take a chance on a guy like me?"

The strangest thought struck me as I stared into his mossy pair of vulnerable eyes: Bradley was just as nervous and insecure as me. That meant something in my fear of not being liked, or worry over not being good enough, was universal. Bradley felt it too. Perfect, beautiful, football-player Bradley.

I blinked, struggling to grasp what the thought meant.

It meant that I, Lexie Greene, wasn't the only person who had weaknesses, or fears, or imperfections. Bradley, with his mussed hair, wrinkled pants, love of Arby's—who had just stepped on my toes for the second time—had flaws as numerous as mine. But I still adored him, wanted to be with him.

That also meant that I, the imperfect, size 12–14 Lexie Greene, was still lovable. And, if what Bradley had just said meant anything at all, Bradley *did* like the occasionally-blemished Lexie Greene. My heart fluttered in my chest.

I was good enough for anyone just being Lexie Greene.

That single moment and lone realization changed everything. I shook my head, coming out of my reverie in time to notice a note of panic come into Bradley's eyes. We'd stopped dancing and stood in the middle of the small courtyard, staring at each other in silence.

"I mean . . . take your time to decide of course. Didn't mean to, uh, rush you or anything," he stammered. "You don't have to answer now or—"

"Oh!" I cried, realizing he wrongly interpreted my silence. "No, I'm sorry Bradley. That's not it at all. I just realized that I'm . . . I'm good enough."

His eyes narrowed. "I'm sorry . . . I'm a bit lost. Am I supposed to—"

I laughed, leaning back. "I just . . . I never realized it, and it's the first time and . . . it's so wonderful! I've always thought that I had to be perfect, or a size eight, or able to wear a bikini before I'd be worthy of someone, but that's not the case, is it? We like people in spite of their weaknesses."

"No," he said. "I'm not sure what a size eight even looks like. But I think you're perfect."

"Oh, this is wonderful!" I said, grabbing his hands. "Bradley, of *course* I want to, how did you say it? *Thumbs up, let's do this?*"

"Ha! This is why I think you're perfect." His face dropped, sobering instantly. "But are you sure, Lexie? I don't want you to feel pressured or anything. I'm not perfect. I'm really *not* perfect."

I felt so light and free I wanted to throw my arms around him, but I squeezed his hands instead. Never in my life had I comprehended that I could be loved despite my flaws, but now it seemed so clear. Why hadn't I realized it before?

"No pressure," I reassured him. "I promise. I've never wanted anything more."

He lifted a hand to my chin, propping it just underneath my jaw to tilt my face up so I saw his beautiful eyes.

"Boston Cream Pie is my favorite cake, which doesn't make any sense at all," he said. "I hate cooking, so I often buy DiGiorno's and Ben and Jerry's. Krispy Kremes and I have a love affair that's a little scandalous, to be honest, and at my heaviest I weighed 270. Lexie Greene, I am not perfect either."

I swallowed. "I know."

Our faces were only a few inches apart. I could feel the soft caress of his breath on my cheek. I wanted to lean into him and never go away, to feel the heavy wrap of his solid arms around me. My eyes fluttered closed and seconds later I felt the warm press of his soft lips against mine. He pulled me close, wrapping an arm around my shoulder. I fell into him, and the sensation took my breath away, leaving tingles running up and down my spine.

"That," he whispered when he pulled away, "is something I've wanted to do since the day I met you at the pub."

I laughed, and we entwined our hands, and together we, two imperfect people, danced under the bright lights and rumbling sky.

Chapter 53—Promise and Light

"Shut. Up."

Megan stared at me from across her farm-fresh egg omelet with nitrate-free bacon, her mouth agape and eyes wide.

"I'm serious!" I said, laughing and stirring my kale smoothie with a straw. "Then he kissed me."

"Under twinkle lights?"

"Yes, under twinkle lights."

She leaned forward. "I can't believe you had your first kiss under twinkle lights. That's incredible. Is your life a movie? What does this mean for you guys? Are you dating now? Is he still here?" She looked around, as if Bradley could be waiting in the corner of the tiki hut. "Can I meet him? He sounds too good to be true."

"He already went back to school, but yeah. We are dating now. We're going to try long-distance and see how it goes."

Megan flipped her long brown hair over her shoulder and leaned back with a dreamy sigh, her plate of protein forgotten despite her complaints of being ravenous after a difficult workout.

"What a lovely story you and Bradley have. Speaking of, have you heard about the internship yet?"

I shook my head.

"What if you don't get it?"

"Then I'll just find another one and keep applying. I'm still early in the game, but it was such a great chance that I didn't want to pass it up. I should hear soon."

Megan smiled. "I'm so happy for you, Lexie. You deserve a really great guy and a great internship, so I'll keep my fingers crossed that they both work out."

My eyes narrowed on her, uncomfortable with speaking so much about myself. "What about you? Still riding the troubled dating waters?"

She shrugged with a wry smile. "I'm always treading bad dating waters. I'm getting used to it by now."

"No prospects?"

"There was one," she said, sipping at a cool glass of water. "But he ended up having this weird fetish for glitter that I couldn't get past, and he was always calling his mom. He called her once to help him make a decision on what kind of pizza to buy."

Both of us grimaced, but ended up laughing.

"Hey, listen, I've been meaning to ask you a question," I said after finishing the last of my morning smoothie with a loud slurp. "Would you be interested in joining the *Health and Happiness Society*? Mira and Bitsy and I are hoping to infuse it with a little bit of life. We're still getting together but we want . . . I don't know . . . something fresh. Bitsy thought you could teach us a little bit about weight lifting."

She brightened. "Really? I think I'd like that. Weekly meetings, right?"

I nodded. "Yeah, and Bitsy's kind of a drill sergeant, so you'll probably like her."

"Maybe it will help me have more motivation." Her shoulders slumped. "I'm losing my mojo."

The idea of Megan losing mojo seemed so foreign that I didn't even know what to say at first, but the alarm on my phone buzzed, reminding me that I had one other thing to do before classes started. I silenced it.

"I need to get going," I said, gathering my things together. "The *Health and Happiness Society* meets tonight. Want to come?"

She grinned. "Definitely."

"Great, I'll text you the details." I stood, hesitating. "Listen, Megan, I just want you to know that I appreciate you and your friendship. You've been such a good friend, and you've helped me start to learn who I am. I don't think I could put a price on how much that means."

She waved a hand through the air. "Aw, Lexie. You just needed to see how awesome you were, that's all. We've all been there at some point. My mom helped me out of my slump, and now you'll help someone else out of theirs."

I smiled. "Yeah, but thanks for helping me out of mine."

With one last wave I headed out the door.

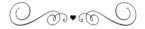

The last time I'd stopped at the cemetery, I'd been angry, hurt, and confused. Now I quietly walked through the rows of graves and headstones, taking in the warm heat of summer and fresh green grass, with a new kind of stillness in my heart.

"Hey, Dad," I said, sitting next to his headstone. I leaned back on my palms and stretched my legs out, clad in the first-ever pair of yoga pants that I'd worn with pride. The way the snug black material fit my legs felt more like a hug than a judgment now. I wore them all the time.

"I came to tell you that I'm not mad at you anymore. I'm actually . . . I'm just grateful for you. I'm grateful for all that I've learned. And I wish we could have had a different lifestyle so you could be here to meet Bradley, or to have seen Kenzie in her wedding dress, but I can't change the past. I can, however, change the future. And that's what I've done."

I hesitated, swallowing back a thick knot of emotion. A few birds twittered by, the only company I had in the calm tranquility of the graveyard.

"I'm dating Bradley now. I'm still counting calories and exercising, but I'm not so obsessed. In fact, I haven't weighed in . . . I don't know how long." I stared into the distance, thinking over the past six months. "Everything is so different now. Mom and I are getting along better, though we aren't perfect. Kenzie and I are actually acting like sisters. And, while I miss you, it doesn't hurt as much as it used too."

Although Dad didn't answer me back, and I felt no whisper of wind to indicate he was near, the way it always happened in the movies, I knew that he was proud of me. It welled up in my chest, spilling out my eyes in hot tears. Dad was proud of me, and *I* was proud of me.

"I love you, Dad. And, most important of all, I finally love me."

I lingered a few minutes, taking in the warm dance of sunlight across my dappled skin. The future hovered in front of me, uncertain, but filled with light. I couldn't wait to head toward it, to meet in the evening with my friends, and video chat with Bradley before bed. It seemed that life had never been so full of promise before.

And neither had I.

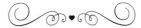

August 15th

Dear Miss Greene,

Delta Publishing is pleased to inform you that your application for the two-month publishing internship has been accepted. Enclosed is the information packet, complete with required paperwork, that we ask you fill out and return as soon as possible. We will be in touch with further details once the formal contract has been signed.

Thank you for your application. We look forward to working with you.

Sincerely,

Debbie Maughn

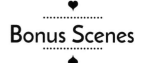

Bonus Scenes

♥

The Best Surprise Ever

♠

The smell of popcorn filled the air with a delicious, buttery zing.

Rachelle and I waded through a crowd of people thronging the Eagles' college football stadium, navigating around oversized hands, painted faces, and the occasional scream from an already-drunk frat boy. A fresh breeze of crisp fall air poured in from the portals leading to the football field. My stomach growled when we passed a pretzel stand. I hadn't eaten since breakfast that morning when we left home.

"What if Bradley's not that excited to see me?" I asked, biting my nails. "Maybe I shouldn't surprise him at one of his football games."

Rachelle rolled her eyes.

"You're kidding, right? I mean, you have met Bradley before? You do know how much he likes you."

The truth behind her reassuring words didn't quell the self-conscious feeling rising from deep in my chest. Bradley and I had been officially dating for several months now, but I'd had yet to meet his daily friends. What if he wasn't excited to see me? What if he hated surprises? Turns out Megan hates surprises. I'd found that out the hard way on her birthday. I dodged two young boys darting through the crowd and headed for portal K.

"It's just that he hasn't introduced me to his friends yet," I pointed out. "Maybe he doesn't want me to meet them."

The words stuck in my throat. *Maybe he's just a little bit ashamed of me.* Showing up this way could be forcing him into something he didn't want.

"I'm new to this relationship thing," I muttered, annoyed with my rampant insecurities. Bradley and I didn't get to spend a lot of time together, so meeting up with him again riled my nerves. "I don't really know how it works."

"You met his friends the first time you met him, remember?"

I thought back to the night at Lucky's Irish Pub with a sigh. "Yeah, but that was an accident. Neither of us had known the other would be there."

235

"Get over it, Lexie. He adores you and you know it. You've never come out here before. That's why. Not because he's ashamed of you. Besides, you look super hot. Are those the new jeans that Kenzie helped you pick out?"

My hands wandered to my hips, covered by the first size-twelve pants that I'd ever been able to comfortably wear. They felt glorious. How perfect that I should see Bradley the first time I wore them? Too perfect. Sliding into them that morning felt like victory. Getting into a size-twelve had been hard. The less weight I had to lose—and the more fitness I achieved in the meantime—meant that consistent loss came slower, and at a greater price. Bitsy moaned about it almost weekly at our meetings.

"Here's portal K," I said, glancing to the two tickets that Bradley's roommate Chris had sent me. "We're on row 12."

"Forget our seats. Let's buy a Slurpee!" Rachelle cried, licking her lips as we passed another snack stand. I grabbed her arm and pushed her ahead of me. If I didn't get a hold of her now, I'd probably lose her until the end of the game. We stumbled into the bright sunlight together. The beginning strains of the marching band warming up echoed through the stadium. Memories of Dad caught me by surprise. He had loved college football, and we'd often gone together.

"So how is this going down again?" Rachelle asked, plopping onto her plastic seat once we'd found it. "After the game you're going to surprise Bradley outside the locker room?"

"Yeah. Chris told me where to wait when he sent me the tickets."

"And you're sure Bradley doesn't know?"

"Chris said he didn't."

A delicious tingle zipped down my spine. It had been over six weeks since he'd been out to see me in his junky old car. Most of our relationship had occurred over Skype, so the thought of not only seeing him, but being able to touch him, made me tingly with excitement. Rachelle popped a handful of caramel corn in her mouth.

"Maybe I'll hang out with Chris, then," she said. "Do you know him well?"

"No. Never met him."

Rachelle skimmed the field. "He certainly got us good enough seats. Is he single?"

"Perpetually, I hear. Kind of a player."

Her eyes lit up. "Just my type."

Chris had snagged us seats in the lower sections instead of the nosebleed, not far above the Eagles' sideline. I'd have several glimpses of Bradley through the game.

And oh, how I hoped he'd be excited to see me.

A swelling cheer broke through the student section when the band started up and the announcer came overhead. Out of one of the tunnels leading onto the field streamed the Eagles football team through an arch of purple and white balloons. My breath caught when I recognized Bradley's thick shoulders—which appeared even bigger beneath the shoulder pads—in the midst of the many players. The number 34 filled his back.

"Oh, hello number 67!" Rachelle called, looking at the field through a set of small binoculars. She smacked me with the back of her hand without taking her eyes away. "Lexie, did you see him? His legs are bigger than tree trunks. He could probably bench press me!"

The game started with a frenzy of energy. I spent most of my time watching the back of Bradley's head instead of the game. By halftime, the Eagles had pulled ahead by twenty-one points. Just before the second half started, Bradley's face flashed up on the mega TV screen while he spoke with one of the coaches. His hair was a disheveled mess of half curls. Streaks of black ran across his cheeks below his eyes. A cheer rose from the crowd when he and several others jogged onto the field. My heart fluttered.

That handsome football player was all mine. Assuming, of course, he wanted to see me. Despite knowing Bradley cared for me, I couldn't get rid of the niggling of doubt. It plagued me for the rest of the game.

What if?

"Let's just hang out here while the crowd thins," Rachelle said when the game ended. She sat back in her chair. "Then you can go meet Bradley, and I will find Mr. 67. I think he needs a date tonight."

Waiting outside the locker room felt like standing on a bed of sharp nails. No matter how I distracted myself, nothing helped. At first, no one came out.

"What if we waited too long?" I asked, fidgeting with the bottom of my jacket sleeves. "What if he's already gone? This whole thing will be ruined."

But then his face can't fall in disappointment when he sees me.

"Just relax. It always takes them awhile to come out. It's only been thirty minutes since the end of the game. Hopefully he's showering."

Rachelle lounged against the wall behind me, chewing on the end of a straw. When the locker room door open, she straightened. The beefy number 67 strode out alone, his ham-like arms swinging from side to side.

"Hello evening entertainment," she sang under her breath. Without a backward glance to me, Rachelle started after him. "See ya, Lexie. Call you later."

She fell into stride with Mr. 67 just before he reached the parking lot. He looked down at her, but whatever she said must have captured his attention, because he didn't try to run away. They disappeared, leaving me alone.

A dangerous thing considering my nervous state of mind.

"It's Bradley," I said, biting my bottom lip. "He'll definitely be excited. Definitely. No problem."

My false sense of confidence did nothing to quiet the insecure voices insisting he wouldn't be happy. *You've never been in a relationship before,* they whispered. *It opens you up for all kinds of pain and vulnerability.*

Why couldn't I just enjoy this moment?

Another interminable ten minutes passed. Various football players left in pairs or by themselves. A familiar head of dark brown hair and broad shoulders stepped out, bags slung over his arms and resting at his side. My heart skipped a beat. Bradley.

He laughed at something another player said, nodding a farewell when the two split ways. Luckily, Bradley veered to the left, heading my direction while fishing in his pocket. When he pulled out his phone, I hesitated.

What if?

I could still back out. Turn around. Hide my face. He'd never have to know. Unless Chris told him, of course. Then came the not-so-small-matter of wrangling Rachelle off her date. No, I had no choice. I had to face the possibility of rejection or mortal embarrassment.

"Hey," I called, though my voice sounded strangled. "Bradley?"

His head snapped up as he heard his name. He stopped walking. I held my breath, feeling as if the blood in my veins had frozen. What would he do? Would his face fall in disappointment? Would he see me then act like he hadn't? The slow-as-molasses smile that I loved slowly slipped across his face.

"Lex?"

A breath of relief escaped me.

"Hey."

"Get over here, girl. I was just about to call you!"

He dropped his bags and spread his arms. Without hesitating, I closed the distance between us with just a few steps, running into his hard-as-steel chest. He picked me up and spun me around, wrapping his warm arms all the way around my back.

"You're crazy!" he cried. "What are you doing here? This is the best surprise ever."

"Chris got me tickets. He helped me out to surprise you." My breath caught for just a moment. "I hope that's al—"

He set me down, grabbed my face, and planted his lips on mine before I could finish my response. I grabbed his shoulders, flooded with a sweet, lightheaded rush of energy. When he pulled away, I kissed him again.

"Good grief, girl. It's been too long since I could do that," he said, pressing our foreheads together. "How long are you here? Tell me forever."

"Ha! No. Just the weekend. Rachelle and I have a hotel not too far from here."

He feigned disappointment but kept an arm around my waist. "Good enough. What did you think of the game?"

"I didn't really pay attention," I said with a grin, enjoying the way he kept our faces only inches apart. "I was too busy staring at the tight, attractive butt of number 34."

Bradley rolled his eyes.

"Where's Rachelle?"

"She ran after number 67," I said, glancing to where they'd disappeared near the parking lot. "Said she'd call me later."

"What a lucky coincidence. She'll probably meet up with us at the apartment later. Chris is number 67."

My eyes grew. "Seriously? Chris is 67?"

"Yeah. They'll make an interesting date tonight. But hey, who cares about them? It's just the two of us now, so let's make the best of it. I need food in the worst way. Let's be losers and get take out and head back to my place. I don't think it's too disastrous, anyway. Though I won't make any promises. Chris is kind of a slob."

"Are you sure?" I asked, pulling away to look in his eyes. "You really don't mind me just showing up? You don't have to introduce me to anyone, or any of your friends, or anything like that. I just wanted to see you and—"

He pulled away, holding me by the upper arm. "Are you kidding? I can't wait to introduce you to everyone! I'd take you into the locker room with me, but trust me, there are things that you'd see in there that you can't *un*see. I'd never do that to someone I cared about."

He threaded his fingers through mine, grabbed both of his bags with one hand, and steered me to the parking lot. A sense of relief spread tingles in a little rush through my skin. I squeezed his hand, feeling the glow of being around Bradley again infuse me with a new sense of life.

Of course he'd been excited. Why had I even been worried? I'd been a fool to ever think otherwise.

No, We Are the Best

I hadn't known exactly what to expect from Bradley's apartment. Aside from meeting his friends and viewing his day-to-day life, being able to see his living quarters would tell me a lot about him. Despite my almost fanatical opinion of him, the long-distance aspect of our relationship meant we really didn't know a lot about each other yet. At least, not beyond what Skype could give us.

So the apartment I walked into was nothing like what I'd planned on.

He and Chris lived in a small place—more like a closet—just off campus. Except for two doors leading into separate bedrooms and a third for their bathroom, the rest of the apartment was just one big floor plan with a super-sized TV on one wall and a half kitchen with a three-legged table.

"So . . . uh . . . If I had known you were coming I would have cleaned up a bit," he said, frantically grabbing at discarded wrappers as he walked past. He tossed the Redbox movie we'd rented on the couch and kicked aside a pair of sneakers. "Chris is kind of a slob, like I said."

A stack of old pizza boxes sat on the floor near four crushed soda cans and a complicated remote control. Underneath the disaster of belongings and Twix wrappers hovered the slight stench of dirty socks. An air freshener plugged in nearby covered the room with a faintly floral scent.

"It's . . . charming," I said, venturing in one step at a time.

Bradley swept an armful of old paper plates into a garbage bag before slinging his football bags into a room in the back. I set the brown bag of Chinese takeout on the counter in between an empty box of cake batter and a couple of red Solo cups.

"Sorry," he said, kicking aside a pile of dirty clothes. "I hardly spend any time here. I've tried to get Chris to clean up, but both of us are so busy during the season that we just kind of crash here."

Except for our late-night video chats, I had noticed that a good deal of Bradley's time was spent either at practice or at the library. I didn't wonder why anymore.

"No problem."

I eyed the half-moon table with a hearty amount of skepticism. None of the three chairs clustered around it matched. The missing leg of the table had been replaced with old science fiction novels.

"How about we eat on the couch?" I suggested.

Of the whole apartment, the only clean area that seemed partially safe was the couch. Not even a single breadcrumb littered the smooth surface. I reached out to rub the tips of my fingers on it.

"Leather?" I asked. Bradley rolled his eyes.

"Yeah. It's the only thing that Chris really takes care of around here. He bought it with some money he got when his grandfather died. As you can tell, he's obsessed with movies. He takes the entire experience very seriously, so a clean couch is necessary."

Aside from the massive TV dominating one wall, five CD cases lay open on top of an overturned cardboard box, which I assumed served as a coffee table of sorts. The slots in the cases were chock full of DVDs. They spilled open so wide the zippers wouldn't even close.

"I see."

"We can eat on the couch," he said, tossing a few more empty pop bottles in a garbage bag. "Let me just . . . uh . . . find something to eat on."

I picked up a few bits of garbage, stuffing them inside the white bag he'd been patrolling the apartment with, while Bradley scrounged through the kitchen. I didn't dare ask if they had plates. Two of the open cupboards lay bare except for a package of ramen noodles and salt. My quest took me closer to Bradley's room. He'd left the light on, illuminating a room far different than the rest of the apartment. The sounds of him shuffling around behind me continued, so I pressed the door open with the tips of my fingers and stepped inside.

While not perfect, his quarters were a vast improvement. No trash littered the floor. His covers had been thrown to the top of the bed in what must have been a fast attempt to make it before he left. Most of his clothes hung in the closet, and four pairs of shoes clogged the closet floor. On top of his desk sat a large, framed picture. I picked it up.

Bradley had his arms around two girls that looked slightly younger than him. Their brown hair and crinkled eyes indicated they were definitely his sisters. Behind them stood an older man with a severe expression, compressed lips, and salt-and-pepper hair. A middle-aged woman with a smile and a face that could have been Bradley's twin stood next to him. Bradley's parents, no doubt.

"That was taken before I came to college," he said from just behind me. I jumped, but he grabbed the photo before I dropped it. "My two younger sisters almost look like twins, don't they?"

"You have a beautiful family. Sorry, I didn't mean to be snooping, or anything."

He waved it off and flopped onto his bed, stacking his hands behind his head.

"Have a look around. I have nothing to hide."

The lines around his eyes gave him a tired appearance, no doubt exhausted from the game. But since I was finally in his bedroom, and he extended the invitation, I continued looking around. Most of the walls were bare except for a few pictures, placed in random array by someone who clearly didn't have any sense of organization in mind. Behind his door hung a peg filled with jackets. The fishy smell of the kitchen didn't seep in here, and the same floral scent that covered the rest of the apartment dominated here.

I sat on the edge of the bed next to him. He shrugged and put a hand on my knee.

"Do you like living here?"

"Chris is fine, but I'm normally out at practice, a game, class, or whatever else."

"Speaking of your game, let's go eat. You look exhausted."

He saluted. "Yes ma'am."

"Mind if I use the bathroom first?" I asked as he stood up and headed for the hallway.

"No! Wait!" He grabbed my shoulder to stop me. "Let me check it first."

I nodded. "Ah, yes. Good plan."

While the sounds of him scrubbing a toilet and throwing more clothes into Chris's room came from the bathroom, I set out the food on the cardboard box and pulled it near the couch. We'd rented a comedy from Redbox, but the sheer amount of technology along the back wall frightened me, so I left it for him to deal with. He came out of the bathroom a little while later.

"All good."

When I came back out, the previews for the movie played across the big screen, and Bradley waited on the couch, his forearms leaning on his upper thighs. He waved two forks in one hand.

"No plates," he said. "We must have run out."

"You don't own any plates?"

He shook his head. "Chris doesn't really cook. Or do dishes. So we make it a lot easier for ourselves. You good with just this?" He motioned to the takeout containers.

"Yeah," I said, grabbing the fork. "Thanks."

He fluffed up his fried rice, slipping me a glance out of the corner of his eyes. "You sure? Because it turns out I'm not really that good at planning dates."

"This was a surprise," I said, opening the sweet and sour chicken container. "Nothing for you to plan."

"Seems like most of our dates dwindle into something that's not very romantic," he said, snatching a piece of chicken from my box with a quick smile. "I'm afraid I'm not very good at that kind of thing. Sorry."

I shrugged. "Me either. I think takeout and a comedy is perfect."

He leaned over and planted a kiss on my cheek. "Thanks, Lexie. You're the best. Seriously."

A flash of warmth covered my heart in a warm blanket. I smiled at him.

"No. *We* are the best."

Makeup Death Trap

"**Are you sure** you want to do this?" Rachelle asked quietly, her lips pushed to one side of her face, eyes following Kenzie as she flitted around the kitchen. "Shopping with Kenzie is brave enough, but shopping for makeup with Kenzie? Look at her. She's fluttering around like a fairy."

The tone of Rachelle's voice said it all: I'd just walked into a death trap.

"It's for her wedding," I said in an equally quiet voice, shifting uncomfortably. "She wants to figure out what she's going to do with her makeup. I'm the maid of honor. I can't just abandon her because I feel awkward about it."

"Well, technically, you could," Rachelle drawled, grabbing her purse from the couch. "But it wouldn't be very nice. Good luck." She glanced over her shoulder when Kenzie started to hum a Mariah Carey song. "I think you're going to need it."

Kenzie flounced up just as Rachelle left. "Let's go!" she cried, peanut butter and jelly sandwich wedge in hand. Her purse jangled as she bounced. "I'm so excited!"

Kenzie had always been blessed with the ability to entertain herself by talking, which meant I had free reign to let my thoughts slide by as we drove to the mall five minutes later.

"Smokey eyes," she said, finishing off the last of her sandwich. "That's what I'm going to have her try on me first. We'll take pictures of everything she does, and then if we really like something, we'll buy everything she used. Everything!"

She clapped while stopped at a red light.

"Isn't being a girl so fun?"

"So fun," I agreed blandly, but folded my arms in front of me and tried not to dread the upcoming appointment.

Ten minutes later we walked into an austere, pristine department store together. A cloud of different perfumes hit me at the same time.

My nose wrinkled and eyes watered. Kenzie drew in a deep breath and let it all out.

"Ah!" she breathed. "I love the smell of the mall. Come on. I made an appointment for both of us just in case they got busy."

Right across from the main doors waited the makeup and perfume counter, where two salesladies hovered like hawks in navy blue dress skirts.

"Welcome!" A tall redhead with legs that seemed to go on forever stepped forward. "I haven't seen you for a while, Kenz. Where have you been?"

"Ugh." Kenzie moaned. "So busy! Weddings are ridiculously stressful. Don't ever get married, Jennifer. And if you must, just elope."

"Sounds like it's time to do a little makeup pamper session," Jennifer said. She wore a bright red lipstick that made her teeth seem as white as the sun. Her stunning beauty cowed me into silence.

"Definitely!" Kenzie threw herself into a sparkling chrome chair with a white leather seat. "Have a seat, Lex. I've booked Jenn, but we have someone else for you."

A tight smile crossed Jennifer's perfect face.

"Yes, yes, of course. Wanda will be working with you, Leslie."

"Lexie."

"Right, so sorry." She smiled demurely and lifted a hand to motion to another worker. "Wanda!" she called. "Your two o'clock is here."

A plump woman with curly hair came around a counter with a wide, fake smile. The jacket of her navy blue skirt suit flared out at the buttons, which were too tight across her middle. Fortunately, I'd gotten the lesser of two intimidating beauties. Unfortunately, she wore so much makeup it looked like she'd put it on with a plaster knife.

"Hi!" Wanda called, smacking a wad of wintergreen gum beneath her teeth and waving with just her wrist. "I'm Wanda. I'll be doing your makeup today. Are you getting married?"

"Oh, no, just my sister. I'm the maid of honor."

"Congrats!" she squealed. "How fun!"

A defined edge of blush ran along the top of her cheekbone, and although she wore mostly navy blue, tones of bright purple and pink decorated her eyes. Her lashes were so thick and heavy they looked like evergreen branches. Several small jewels sparkled in their thick depths.

"Let's get started." She tapped her finger against her lips, eyes narrowed in scrutiny. "I know *just* what to do. You have a wonderful skin tone, but big pores, so we're going to have go clean you up a bit."

"Great," I muttered, managing a smile. Kenzie and Jennifer—who brandished a cotton swab and made swirling motions with her hands while she told a story—chattered away like a pair of reunited squirrels. Wanda shoved me in a chrome chair and spun me around to face her.

"Do you tweeze?" she asked.

"Tweeze? Uh . . . no. I don't believe so."

"I can tell." Wanda giggled and fluffed her curly hair with one hand. "We've got a little forest going on up here."

"Do it!" Kenzie called. "I'll pay extra if you tweeze her!"

Before I could even protest, Wanda had my head tilted back at an awkward angle, a pair of tweezers in hand, and waves of her wintergreen gum washed over my face as she chewed and chewed and chewed. Each time she pulled out one of my eyebrow hairs, I gave a little squeal.

"Ow!"

Wanda smacked away my hand when I reached up to cover my face. "Nope," she sang. "Just getting started, honey pie. Beauty is pain."

Honey pie?

McKenzie giggled from the seat next to mine, and I silently promised to share my pain with her once we finished.

For the next twenty minutes, I kept my eyes closed and endured the silent ride of horror. Jennifer, Kenzie, and Wanda chatted back and forth, talking about bridesmaids, honeymoons, and the agony of memorizing the names of new in-laws. I dug my fingers in the armrest and braced myself for impact. Based on how much Wanda brushed, dipped, cleaned, wiped, and patted my face, I knew I'd look like a circus clown.

"I think we got it," Wanda said with a long breath. "You're just beautiful."

The sound of her heels clicking as she stepped back to survey her work told me it was safe. I opened my eyes for the first time in almost half an hour. She held up a hand mirror. I jumped back.

"Whoa!"

Whether she had done it on purpose or not, Wanda had just recreated her own face on mine. A line of blush so thick it had a defined line ran along one side of my face. Eye shadow filled the entire space from my eyelashes to my eyebrows in various shades of purple and pink. The eyeliner along the top and bottom of my eye was so thick I should have been on my way to a gothic poetry reading.

"Well?" Wanda asked with a crazy shine in her eyes, as if she were already imagining how to make it as full as her own. "What do you think?"

I swallowed. *I look like a freak show.*

"I . . . I don't have any words," I whispered. Wanda beamed.

"I know, right? It's amazing what can be done with the right amount of makeup. That blush is just perfect. Really brings out those cheekbones. Not to mention how much more feminine you look with two defined eyebrows. They really do make or break the face."

Kenzie stared at me in wide-eyed horror. Even Jennifer, who stood behind her, hadn't said anything. Wanda continued explaining all the different colors she'd used and why, chattering without regard to our horror.

"Well, bride-to-be?" Wanda asked, turning to Kenzie with a wide grin. "What do you think?"

Both Jennifer and Kenzie dropped their horrified expressions, replacing them with awkward smiles.

"It's . . . it's apparent that you have talent," Kenzie said, swallowing. "I think this gives us a wonderful idea of what we . . . want for the wedding."

Jennifer's eyes narrowed. "It looks really good, Wanda. You're improving, definitely. But I'm thinking that purple eye shadow won't go as well with the bright pink. What do you think, Kenzie?"

"Yes, definitely," she said instantly.

Wanda tilted her head to one side, as if considering. "Yes," she eventually agreed, reaching for a fresh piece of gauze. "I think you're right. I'll redo it."

"No!" I cried, leaping upright. "I-I just mean that this is . . . perfect. I don't want you to undo anything. Now we know we won't use purple. Right, Kenz?" I asked through gritted teeth.

Kenzie smiled with easy, natural, beauty, looking like a Greek goddess that had just bestowed herself on the world. Whatever exploded on my face after Wanda's ministrations belonged in a circus. At least Bradley lived six hours away so I knew I wouldn't run into him.

"Right. Thank you, Wanda. You've been very helpful," Kenzie said, her lips pressed together and trembling with suppressed laughter. "I really appreciate the help."

Wanda popped her gum a few times, played with my hair and smiled. "So welcome!"

She spun on her heel and headed to the counter where a customer had just walked up. Kenzie's restraint lasted until Wanda slipped out of earshot. She doubled over and burst into laughter. Jennifer surveyed me with an amused gaze full of pity.

"Oh, Lexie!" Kenzie cried. "You look *horrible.*"

Hearing the words from her lips eased my fears. My greatest worry had been Kenzie's approving the ridiculous look, because then I'd have to look like a drag queen for the wedding, and wedding photos last forever.

"Wanda goes a little crazy," Jennifer said with a sigh. She held a Q-Tip like a cigarette in between her fingers. Her lips twitched in a slow drawl. "I should have warned you, but it always turns out so funny that I couldn't help myself. I needed a good laugh. Thanks for being a good sport, and don't worry. I go to a girl named Terry that can take care of you. You'll love her, and she certainly didn't learn makeup at the circus."

Despite my annoyance, all three of us fell into a rolling laugh. Spending time with Kenzie never went the way I wanted it, but it felt great to have a sister.

♥
The Massage Table
♠

"**Congratulations on getting** the internship!" Rachelle cried, chewing on a straw from her 44-oz Sonic limeade. "I signed us up for a massage!"

She spread her arms, indicating the brown brick building in front of us. A slip of paper sat in my hand. *Good For One Free Massage* ran across the front. Below that sat the date with an appointment five minutes away written on it. My stomach roiled.

"A massage?"

Rachelle rolled her eyes. "Don't be such a wimp. Getting a massage is a lot of fun. You'll love it, I promise. I come every month."

I'd never disrobed in front of anyone before. Lying naked on a table in front of a stranger didn't sound like my idea of fun.

"But—"

"It's the naked thing, isn't it?" She slammed her car door shut. "They're professionals, Lexie. Don't worry about it. They've seen all kinds of bodies. Plus, they don't care. Look at me! I go all the time and no one has ever said a word!"

The hot summer sun rolled off the asphalt and pavement in long, sultry waves, distorting the air. The heat of the melting tar baked through the bottom of my flip-flops. Reluctantly, I followed behind her, dragging my feet as I went. No matter how confident or at ease Rachelle might be with her plus-sized body, that didn't mean I cared for other people getting a full view of my flabby legs, regardless of whether I had lost weight or not. A cool, air-conditioned breeze hit me in the face when we stepped into a small waiting room swathed in calming lights. Soft, harp-like music played in the background. A waterfall trickled down the wall to the right.

"See?" Rachelle asked, holding her hands up to gesture around. "Doesn't it smell divine? I could live here. I asked them if they'd let me spend the night once, but it was a no."

I pulled in a breath of lavender.

"Yeah, smells great. But I still don't know—"

250

Rachelle grabbed my wrist and pulled me farther in. "You need to do more new stuff, Lex. I'm your best friend. It's my obligation to pull you out of your comfort zone. C'mon, just trust me. No one is going to care what you look like, and you don't have to get totally naked if you don't want. Although I suggest it. There's something very freeing about a full body massage."

She stepped up to the front desk to check us in. A young, blonde worker with full lips dressed in black brought me a glass of ice water with a lemon wedge. I thanked her with a nervous smile, avoiding her eyes. Would she be the one to see me naked? What a nightmare! I wouldn't do it. No *way* would I let someone that young and beautiful see my rolling love handles.

By the time Rachelle came back from checking us in, I'd nearly worked myself into a nervous fit.

"Rachelle, I'm not sure I can do this. I'm too nervous and—"

"You'll be fine. I had them give you Marjorie. She's wonderful, and she'll put you right at ease."

"Marjorie? You're chummy with the people that work here or something?"

She snorted and plucked a sesame cracker from a sideboard that offered healthy snacks. A small bowl of grapes, a pile of olives, and chilled pear slices sat next to them. "I come here at least once a month. Professional massages are one of the only things that relax me."

Rachelle did seem tense lately, though she wouldn't tell me why. I had an idea that she'd encountered some boy problems, or worse, a *lack* of boy problems, but she'd always been a closed book. I never pushed her. For all her bright laughter, audacious flirting, and outrageous attention tactics, Rachelle was as closed as vault.

"Lexie?"

A woman in her early thirties stood in a doorway off to the left. She wore the same black outfit that the rest of the employees wore. A belt looped around her waist with a bottle of lotion hanging off her hip. She had a calm, maternal air when she smiled.

"My name is Marjorie. I'll be your masseuse today."

Not knowing what to do with the glass of water, I clutched it in one hand, swallowed back the nervous lump in my throat, and followed. Rachelle waved.

"Just relax!" she called to my back. "It'll be great!"

Marjorie walked a few steps ahead of me into the back hall of the spa. Shoots of bamboo and more tinkling waterfalls decorated the walls, which had dimmed lights. Despite the calming atmosphere, I couldn't relax.

"Is this your first time?" she asked, twisting slightly to look over her shoulder. I nodded, unable to choke any words out. She smiled as if she'd seen it all before. "Then we'll get you settled and comfortable, don't worry."

I'm just going to be naked, lying on a table, in front of a total stranger who might laugh at how imperfect my love handles and cottage cheese thighs look. That's all. Just settle right in, Lexie.

Yeah, I'd surely be really *comfortable.*

She stopped at a room on the left and motioned me inside. A single bed, draped in sheets and a blanket, waited with down-turned sheets. The soft noises of a storm pattered in the background through the speakers on the ceiling. Marjorie reached over and dimmed the lights even further, casting a late-evening glow in the room. At least the lights wouldn't glare and shine over every flaw on my body.

"I can take that water, if you want," she said and held out a hand.

"Oh, thanks. I didn't even realize I still had it."

She set it aside and clasped her hands in front of her. "What kind of pressure are you comfortable with?"

"None."

"None?"

"I mean . . . I don't know." I shook my head. "I . . . what do you normally do? What do you mean by pressure? Because Rachelle's putting a lot of pressure on me to do this, and I'm not that . . ."

I trailed off, realizing she meant something totally different. Unbothered, and likely amused, she smiled in a kind way. To my surprise, it put me at ease. Marjorie didn't seem so bad. She wasn't a devastatingly beautiful young girl with perky boobs and the body of a gazelle.

It helped.

"I'll start with a medium massage pressure, and you can tell me if it's too much or too little." She pulled the sheet farther down. "We're going to start with you lying on your stomach. I'll do a full body massage from there. Are there any sensitive areas or places you want me to avoid?"

All of them! I wanted to scream. Would it be weird to ask her to just massage my neck and arms the whole time? That way I could keep most my clothes on.

"Uh, no," I said. "At least, I . . . uh . . . I don't think so."

Marjorie reached out and put a hand on my arm. "It's okay to be a little nervous. The first massage is new, but I can promise that I'll do everything I can to make you comfortable."

Her reassurance calmed some of my internal panic.

"Sorry. I just . . . I'm just quite shy, really, and I've recently lost a lot of weight but I'm still nervous about my body and—"

"Trust me, Lexie, I've met a lot of people and seen a lot of bodies. No one is perfect, and to be quite honest, your size doesn't matter. My goal is to give you a relaxing massage, that's all."

Her reassurance worked. I let out a long breath.

"Okay . . . thanks."

"Undress to your level of comfort," she said, taking a step back. "You can leave your bra and underwear on if you like. I'll give you a few minutes and then knock before I come back in."

She disappeared with the slight click of the door. While she'd calmed the internal fires of terror welling up inside me, the fear of being laughed at, of my imperfections, my flaws being uncovered for all the world to see, remained. I stared at the bed with a lingering sense of trepidation.

"Why is this so hard?"

Not even the soothing music or the hint of lemongrass in the air made me feel any better. I thought of Rachelle, and how easily things like this came for her. How Megan wouldn't have even hesitated, and could probably elaborate on all the ways that a massage would be beneficial and healthy. My fingers curled into my palms in a tight little fist.

I am a swan with swanitude. I can do this.

I could leave, of course. I didn't have to do the massage. But when would I do it? When would I have the courage if I didn't have it now?

After sucking in a deep breath, I whisked out of my clothes before I lost my nerve, tossed them into a ball on a chair in the corner, and slipped under the sheets face down. The warmth of the bed surprised me. Finally managing to get the sheet pulled up to my shoulders, I laid my head into the head pillow at the top and let out a long breath. Only a few minutes passed before Marjorie knocked on the door, and I answered for her to come in.

"Feeling comfortable?"

"Yes," I said, hearing the surprise in my own voice. "I am, actually."

With my face down, preventing me from seeing her facial expressions or judgment, perhaps the massage wouldn't be so bad.

"I'm going to use a little aromatherapy to help you relax," she said, and I heard the clinking of a couple of bottles near the cupboard. Seconds later, the scent of lemongrass filled my nostrils. Against my wishes, my body did relax. Nearly melted into the massage table. After a few shuffling, squirting noises, she pressed her hands into the muscles of my back with a firm pressure.

Heavenly.

Within minutes under her expert, gentle hands, all my reservations faded away. No comments on back fat, no names, no judgment. She didn't even speak. She just swirled her hands over my back, gliding them over my muscles, kneading in all the right spots, and turning me into a puddle of mush.

She finished an hour later, and I groggily sat up on the table once she left. My skin felt silky and smelled like lemongrass. By the time I'd managed to use my jelly-like muscles and get dressed, I'd started to come out of the relaxed coma. When I opened the door, Marjorie waited outside, a fresh glass of water in hand and a knowing smile on her face.

"How did that feel?" she asked.

Wonderful, I thought.

The feeling of relaxation, even euphoria, had less to do with Marjorie's obvious talent, but everything to do with the freedom of doing something new. Although I'd been afraid, I'd conquered a fear that I'd never even known I had. I, Lexie Greene, the girl who used to hide behind sweat pants and hoodies, had just gotten a massage.

With a smile I took the glass of water. "It was more than I could have ever hoped for," I said, and followed her into the foyer.

♥
....
About the Author
♠

Katie Cross is a big fan of cookies and sweet potatoes. If she's not writing, you can find her weight lifting, trail running with her husband and two vizslas, or drooling over food blogs. Connect with Katie Cross and more of the *Health and Happiness Society* at www.healthandhappinesssociety.com, or visit her YA fantasy stories, *The Network Series*, at www.MissMabels.com.

♥
....
Read more from Katie Cross
♠

Manufactured by Amazon.ca
Bolton, ON

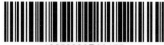

12858392R00155